Updates on Foreign Body in ENT Practice

Edited by Balwant Singh Gendeh

Published in London, United Kingdom

Updates on Foreign Body in ENT Practice
http://dx.doi.org/10.5772/intechopen.1002572
Edited by Balwant Singh Gendeh

Contributors
Amnah Khalid, Balwant Singh Gendeh, Bojan Marinkovic, Dragan Stojanov, Dusan Milisavljevic, Emilia Nissa Khairani, Hardip Singh Gendeh, Jacky Munilson, Melpomeni Bizhga, Milan Stankovic, Muhammad Perwaiz, Natalija Milisavljevic, Nikola Djordjevic, Sameeksha Mishra, Sasa Zivaljevic, Sudhakar Vaidya, Toma Kovacevic, Varun tej Gonuguntla, Yan Edward

First published in London, United Kingdom, 2024 by IntechOpen
IntechOpen is the global imprint of INTECHOPEN LIMITED, registered in England and Wales, registration number: 11086078, 167-169 Great Portland Street, London, W1W 5PF, United Kingdom

For EU product safety concerns: IN TECH d.o.o., Prolaz Marije Krucifikse Kozulić 3, 51000 Rijeka, Croatia, info@intechopen.com or visit our website at intechopen.com.

British Library Cataloguing-in-Publication Data
A catalogue record for this book is available from the British Library

Updates on Foreign Body in ENT Practice
Edited by Balwant Singh Gendeh
p. cm.
Print ISBN 978-0-85466-737-6
Online ISBN 978-0-85466-736-9
eBook (PDF) ISBN 978-0-85466-738-3

Meet the editor

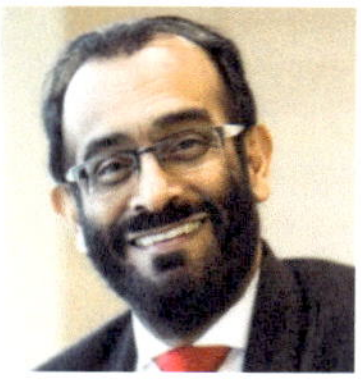

Dr. Balwant Singh Gendeh is a senior consultant ENT surgeon with a subspeciality in rhinology. His previous achievements include being an ENT registrar at the Royal Infirmary, Middlesbrough, UK, in 1993, and a JW Fulbright Scholar to the United States in 1997 at the University of Pittsburgh Medical Center (UPMC), Pittsburgh; Hospital University of Pennsylvania (HUP), Philadelphia; and St Joseph's Hospital, Chicago. He received his diploma from the Fellowship Academy of Medicine Malaysia (FAMM) in 2000. He was the previous board chairman of the Malaysian American Commission on Educational Exchange (MACEE), an international fellow of the American Academy of Otolaryngology—Head and Neck Surgery (AAOHNS), and a fellow of the Academy of Sciences Malaysia (FASc). Dr Gendeh has published 98 scientific papers and 39 book chapters and has edited 11 books.

Contents

Preface

This book discusses selected topics on foreign body in ENT practice, providing insight into advancements in its management. This book includes 6 chapters organized into 3 sections

Section 1

- Current Approach to Diagnosis and Treatment of Foreign Body in Otorhinolaryngology
- Foreign Bodies in ENT in Pediatric Age Group
- Perspective Chapter: Classification and Complications of Aerodigestive Button Batteries and Magnets

Section 2

- Foreign Body in the Airway
- Foreign Bodies in Lower Airways in Children 1–3 Years Old

Section 3

- Foreign Body in the Ear

I would like to take this opportunity to thank and congratulate the chapter authors for their excellent contributions and the valuable time taken to prepare the manuscript. I also thank my valuable teachers from whom I have gained knowledge throughout the years.

I am most grateful to IntechOpen for conceiving this book project and for inviting me to serve as an editor. Thanks also goes to Publishing Process Managers Dorian Salatic and Josip Knapic at IntechOpen for guiding me through the publication process and moving the book ahead in a timely fashion. My kind gratitude goes to the technical editors for arranging the book in a uniform format.

I hope this book publication contributes to the global distribution of knowledge of foreign bodies in ENT practice and its applications in this digital era.

I dedicate this book to my spouse, children, and loved ones for all their patience and understanding.

Balwant Singh Gendeh, MBBS (Kashmir), MS (ORL-HNS)UKM, AM (Mal), FAMM, FASc (M'sia), FMSA
Senior Consultant ENT Surgeon (Rhinology—Allergy, Endoscopic Sinus and Skull Base Surgery, Functional and Cosmetic Nasal Surgery),
Pantai Hospital,
Kuala Lumpur, Malaysia

Visiting Professor,
Department of Otorhinolaryngology, Head and Neck Surgery,
Universiti Kebangsaan Malaysia Medical Center,
Kuala Lumpur, Malaysia

Adjunct Professor,
Tailors University Lakeside Campus,
Subang Jaya, Kuala Lumpur

Section 1

ENT Foreign Body

Chapter 1

Current Approach to Diagnosis and Treatment of Foreign Body in Otorhinolaryngology

Dusan Milisavljevic, Milan Stankovic, Nikola Djordjevic, Toma Kovacevic, Sasa Zivaljevic, Dragan Stojanov, Bojan Marinkovic and Natalija Milisavljevic

Abstract

Foreign body (FB) in ENT is a condition frequently seen in, but not exclusive to, the pediatric population. In adults, poor eating habits, loss of dentition, alcohol consumption, and old age are the factors predisposing patients to FB pathology. Foreign bodies can be classified by type and by localization. By type, FB can be broadly classified as organic or inorganic. Special attention must be devoted to batteries. By location, FBs are commonly classified as aural, nasal, pharyngeal, ingested, and aspirated. High level of suspicion is essential for FB diagnosis. Normal physical exam does not exclude FB diagnosis. Frontal and lateral plain radiographs are helpful, but not sensitive in every case. The majority of ingested FB are low risk objects and pass through gastrointestinal tract without causing any problems. Bronchoscopy should be performed whenever there is a reasonable suspicion of aspirated FB. Recurrent or long-standing pulmonary problems warrant FB consideration.

Keywords: foreign body, esophagoscopy, bronchoscopy, button battery, magnet, aspiration, ingestion, ENT

1. Introduction

A foreign body (FB) is "an object in an organ or body cavity that is not normally present" (according to the Agency for Healthcare Research and Quality (AHRQ)—US Department of Health & Human Services). It remains a diagnostic and surgical challenge, even for experienced otolaryngologists. Foreign body in ENT is a condition most commonly seen in, but not exclusive to, the pediatric population. Infants (1–12 months) and toddlers (1–3 years) are at the highest risk. This is due to the children's tendency to explore the world using their mouth, their tendency to eat and play simultaneously, their relatively smaller airway, and their limited ability to differentiate edible from inedible materials. Children also do not have fully developed posterior dentition, nor is their cough reflex mature. Children with behavioral disorders such as ADHD and hyperactivity disorder are further predisposed to FB incidents [1].

In adults, poor eating habits, loss of dentition, alcohol consumption, and old age are the factors predisposing patients to FB pathology. It should be noted that adults presenting with FB must be inspected for underlying pathology, such as some neurological conditions or malignancies [2].

Higher levels of housing instability and material deprivation are associated with more common FB ingestion and more common complications related to FB ingestion. The odds of complications related to FB ingestion are also much higher in children with comorbidities [3].

History can be helpful, but the clinician should not rely on history too much when considering diagnostic approaches. Regarding aural and nasal foreign bodies, parents often witness the actual event or come to a physician after seeing the foreign body in the nose or the ear canal. If these things do not happen, patients will present with nasal/aural discharge and pain due to mucosal swelling. Regarding esophageal FB, aside from witnessing the event, history often consists of sudden-onset dysphagia/aphagia and drooling. Aspirated FBs are almost always accompanied by an initial choking and coughing event. Children who are verbal can often report where the foreign body is sensed.

Radiograph imaging is usually performed when there is a suspicion of FB. However, it has low sensitivity and specificity for nonmetallic objects. A systematic review and meta-analysis of eighteen articles (4178 patients) showed that the sensitivity of chest CT scans in detecting foreign bodies in children was 99%, while the specificity of chest CT scans was 92%. The authors concluded that while CT can be used to help reduce the number of unnecessary rigid bronchoscopies, it should not be a replacement for gold standard bronchoscopy, especially in cases with a clear history and positive symptoms [4].

Any history of witnessed choking accompanied by gagging, coughing, or cyanotic episodes should be investigated further *via* flexible laryngoscopy and bronchoscopy, regardless of radiographic findings.

The first described foreign body extraction was performed by Verduc in 1717 and consisted of a bronchotomy. Bronchotomy remained a procedure of choice for the next one and a half centuries, despite having a higher mortality rate than observation (23%). In 1876, Killian changed the approach by removing a pork bone from the patient's airway using an esophagoscope, giving rise to the era of endoscopy in FB management. The early twentieth century gave rise to modern rigid bronchoscopes. The fiber-optic bronchoscope was first developed in 1967 by Shigeto Ikeda, thus beginning the new era. Today, fiber-optic bronchoscopy is the gold standard for the diagnosis and management of aspirated foreign bodies [5].

Foreign bodies in the ear, nose, and throat can frequently be managed in the emergency department, especially if the patient provides a history consistent with the foreign body and is calm and cooperative during the examination and removal procedures. On the other hand, many studies point to the problem that arises when an unsuccessful attempt at FB removal is made in the emergency department. Namely, the risk of FB removal failure by an ENT specialist increases significantly following a failed prior removal attempt by a non-ENT specialist. Therefore, each case must be carefully evaluated to minimize the odds in this scenario. More difficult cases should always be referred to an ENT specialist [6].

2. Incidence

In the European Union, the yearly incidence of FBs is around 50.000 for children aged 0–14 years. Out of those, around 1% end up being fatal. This makes choking the 4th leading cause of death in children under 5 years [7, 8].

As people's habits change, so do the types of foreign bodies. Nowadays, safety pins and marbles have been replaced with batteries and plastic toy pieces.

The Susy Safe project is the largest registry of FB incidents. It started collecting data in 2007, at first in the EU and later getting reports from other parts of the world. As of March 6, 2023, there are 35,891 cases registered in the database. According to the database, boys are more likely than girls (53 vs. 47%) to present with a foreign body. Most FB incidents happen at home (83%), and most happen in the presence of an adult (72%). The incidence by region was: ear (19%), nose (26%), mouth and esophagus (25%), pharynx and larynx (10%), and tracheobronchial tree (15%). However, one should bear in mind when looking at this statistical data that it is collected by means of reporting on a case-by-case basis. Also, the project started with the collection of only nonfood foreign bodies and only later incorporated food foreign bodies. The proportion may also vary depending on the region because of different cultures and food types [8].

A large retrospective study of 829 patients in 7 years identified the following relative proportions: nose (58.7%), ear (20.2%), mouth/pharynx/tonsil (12.3%), esophagus (6.2%), and laryngotracheobronchial tree (2.4%). The most common FBs by location were beads in the nose (30.8%); beads in the ear (32.1%); fishbones in the mouth, pharynx, or tonsil (56.8%); nuts and peanuts in the laryngotracheobronchial tree (70%); and coin/disc batteries in the esophagus (80.7%) [9].

A big step forward was made in 1979 (Consumer Product Safety Act), which introduced the cylinder test to reduce the risk of choking in children. The cylinder has an inner diameter of 31.7 mm and a truncated askew with an upper dimension of 51.7 mm and a lower dimension of 25.4 mm. Any toy entering the cylinder without pressure is considered unsuitable for children younger than 3 and is legally banned. For all toys intended for children under 3 years old, the batteries must be secured in compartments with screws [10].

3. Classification of foreign bodies

Foreign bodies can be classified by type and by localization.

By type, FB can be broadly classified as organic or inorganic (**Figure A1**). Special attention must be devoted to batteries, as these are the only FBs that require immediate intervention regardless of the anatomic site that they are in. Around 80% of FBs in the upper aerodigestive tract are organic in nature [8].

In general, metallic objects cause minimal inflammatory response, while organic foreign bodies tend to be more irritating to the upper aerodigestive tract mucosa and tend to cause symptoms much earlier. FBs with high starch content can absorb water and enlarge, subsequently causing even bigger obstruction. Some FBs are potentially toxic to the body (lead objects, drug packets) [11].

By location, FBs are most commonly classified as aural, nasal, pharyngeal, ingested, and aspirated FBs. According to the literature, aural and nasal foreign bodies are more common than aspirated or ingested foreign bodies, but this was dealt with more in the previous chapter. There is reporter bias regarding this matter, as the literature on aural and nasal foreign bodies is much scarcer, due to them being much less of a threat to a patient's well-being, and tertiary centers dealing with aspirated and ingested FBs never come into contact with some of the aural and nasal FBs that are removed in the emergency department.

4. Ear foreign bodies

The external auditory canal (EAC), along with the nose, is the most common site of FB encounter. The majority of ear FBs are found in children; however, adults also frequently present with foreign bodies in this region. Children most commonly insert beads, plastic toy pieces, popcorn kernels, and paper. Adults present with cotton pieces from ear swabs and insects [12].

The EAC is a narrow tube of cartilage and bone, lined with perichondrium and periosteum, and overlying skin that is tightly adherent to the surface. The narrow point of the EAC is the bony-cartilaginous junction, the place at which FB can become impacted, which most commonly happens with unsuccessful removals. Most FBs are found lateral to the isthmus. Additionally, the tympanic membrane is at risk of perforation if further displacement of the FB happens [13].

While many FBs can be removed in the emergency department, careful evaluation must be done prior to the first attempt. Non-graspable foreign bodies are better removed by otolaryngologists with fewer complications compared to emergency department staff removal [13, 14]. Other indications for referral include patients with trauma to the canal or tympanic membrane, a foreign body suspected of touching the tympanic membrane, foreign bodies with sharp edges, or unsuccessful removal attempts. Children have narrow external auditory canals and relatively greater amounts of earwax compared to adults. The risk of eardrum damage increases if a foreign body is in its proximity. Because of this, especially if paired with a noncooperative child, general anesthesia is relatively commonly required for aural FB [15]. In most cases, though, FB can be removed as an outpatient procedure using a combination of instruments, most notably suction, alligator forceps, and a right-angled hook [16]. The procedure is done under microscopic visualization with adequate positioning of the patient. Many aural foreign bodies will spontaneously migrate out of the ear. This is what commonly happens with grommets.

A few rules of thumb can be applied when it comes to dealing with aural foreign bodies [17]:

- Batteries require immediate removal.
- If the foreign body is inorganic, then syringing can be a good option.
- If the foreign body is organic matter, it is best to avoid syringing, as the foreign body could swell and make the extraction more difficult.
- If the foreign object is an insect, the patient's head should be tilted so that the ear with the insect is upward. It is usually a good practice to kill the insect using an alcohol or lidocaine solution, unless there is a suspicion that the tympanic membrane is perforated. After a few minutes, the insect is removed like any other FB.

Complications caused by extraction are lacerations and excoriations to the ear canal and rarely tympanic membrane perforation with or without ossicular chain damage [9].

5. Nasal foreign bodies

Commonly encountered in the pediatric population, nasal foreign bodies comprise around ¼ of FB incidents worldwide. The most common items extracted from the nose are beads, paper slices, food particles, and button batteries [8].

Nasal foreign bodies are most frequently located on the floor of the nasal passage, just below the inferior turbinate, or in the upper parts, anterior to the middle turbinate [17].

A nasal foreign body must be considered in any child with unilateral nasal discharge, even without a history of FB. The discharge usually occurs 4 days after the insertion, but with button batteries, discharge occurs immediately [18].

Most of the nasal foreign bodies can be removed in the emergency department, but doing so requires a careful clinical evaluation. Unsuccessful attempts at nasal FB removal may cause physical harm, such as lacerations of the nasal mucosa or nasal mucosa edema, as well as induce or worsen patient or parent anxiety. All of those factors can complicate subsequent removal attempts and sometimes even necessitate the use of general anesthesia, which is a further risk for the patient [19].

Early plain film X-rays should be justified for unwitnessed foreign body insertions, suspected unknown metallic foreign bodies, and disproportionate discharge or pain [20].

Some FBs are inert and can remain in the nasal cavity for a long time, causing no harm or even causing no major symptoms. Other FBs cause mucosal edema and subsequent erosions, ulcerations, and bleeding. Over time, due to chronic inflammation, these FBs absorb minerals, thus hardening and turning into rhinoliths.

Before the FB removal, a decongestant and local anesthetic should be applied to minimize edema and discomfort during the procedure. The commonly used instrument is a hook or a bent Jobson-Horne probe over and behind a foreign body. In around 60% of the cases, a technique referred to as "mothers kiss" can successfully expel the FB in children too small to blow their nose. The technique is performed by sealing the unaffected nostril and blowing the air gently from mouth to mouth. Balloon catheters (Fogarty) can also be placed intranasally behind the foreign body, partially inflated, and pulled out of the nose. In intubated patients, FB can be pushed into the nasopharynx and removed from there [17].

6. Pharyngeal foreign bodies

The pharynx is the most common localization of FB in the adult population [12, 21]. The most common subsite is the palatine tonsil and the lymphoid tissue at the base of the tongue. The most frequent type of FB is, by far, a fish bone, with its one end stuck in the tonsillar crypt.

Removal of pharyngeal FBs is usually done in outpatient settings. Most of these FBs are easily visualized during oropharyngoscopy using a headlight and proper patient positioning. Most of these FBs can be easily grasped using Magill forceps. In rare cases, as with the posterior pole of the palatine tonsil, vallecula, or pyriform sinus, the FB may not be visualized directly. Flexible endoscopes can be used to visualize the FB and extract it using flexible grabbing forceps passed down the instrument channel. In rare circumstances, this removal can require general anesthesia and a rigid endoscopy.

A rare but serious complication regarding pharyngeal foreign bodies is a migrating foreign body. The FB can migrate to the mucosa, to the soft tissue, or even to adjacent organs, forming abscesses and fistulae. A case series describes pharyngeal FBs migrating to the floor of the mouth, tongue, retropharyngeal region, and soft tissues of the neck [22]. One case study even shows migration of the fish bone to the mediastinum [23].

7. Ingested foreign bodies

Foreign body ingestion is a common occurrence in ENT practice. Foreign bodies can pass through gastrointestinal tract without causing any problems (80%) and may need endoscopic extraction (10–20%) or even surgical removal (<1%) [24]. Outcome depends on the nature of the FB, as well as the patient's clinical and anatomical characteristics. In this chapter, we will be discussing esophageal foreign bodies, as the lower parts of the gastrointestinal tract are not within the domain of the ENT specialist.

A majority of patients with FB ingestion are children between 6 months and 3 years of age [25]. At this age, children regularly put foreign objects in their mouths as a mean of exploring the surroundings. By doing so, they sometimes accidentally swallow these objects. The American Association of Poison Control Centers recorded 83,412 FB ingestions in 2022 among all age groups (55,803 in children under 5 years and 7886 in adults above 20 years). There were no recorded fatal outcomes [26]. Most of them were unintentional [26, 27]. However, there is a substantial portion of adult population in which FB ingestion was intentional. Groups that have greater risk of foreign body ingestion are older people and people with gastrointestinal obstruction, intellectual disability, or secondary gain [27–29].

Impaction place of the FB depends on its morphology. The most common place where FBs get lodged are upper esophageal sphincter (70%), followed by aortic notch (20%) and lower esophageal sphincter (10%) [27]. Most commonly ingested FBs are coins, batteries, magnets, pieces of toys, and pieces of food. Button batteries are one of the most dangerous ingested FBs (refer to Section 9. Special considerations) [30].

Patients with esophageal FB can be asymptomatic or can develop dysphagia, odynophagia, FB sensation, hypersalivation, refusal to eat, retrosternal pain, respiratory distress [24, 27]. As in many other instances, detailed anamnesis and physical examination are in order. Witness statements are of great value. It is important to find out when the incident occurred, what is the FB, how many are there, were there any symptoms at the time of ingestion, is it the first time that FB ingestion occurred, has food or drink been ingested since the incident. It is helpful if the similar object as the FB can be presented to the physician. All of this can sometimes be challenging, especially when working with young children and the incident was not witnessed.

Laboratory tests are often unremarkable when a patient is stable [25]. Both anteroposterior and lateral radiographs are strongly suggested whenever there is a suspicion of the FB ingestion, even with asymptomatic patient (**Figure A2**). It gives additional information about the position and the shape of the FB. However, some FBs are radiolucent and cannot be seen on plain radiograph. Recent meta-analysis has showed that radiographs have 58% sensitivity and 94% specificity for detecting upper digestive tract FBs [31]. In some cases, radiographs have 100% positive predictive value (metallic objects) but 0% for others (wooden objects) [24]. CT scans can be used for radiolucent objects [2, 32]. They are particularly helpful when there is a suspicion of FB-related complication [33]. Contrast swallow studies are not routinely recommended, because they can be the cause of increased risk of aspiration in patients with complete obstruction, can delay treatment, and make the extraction of FBs more challenging by impairing visualization [33].

Ingested FB requires emergent (within 2 h) or urgent (within 24 h) endoscopy. Button batteries, sharp-pointed objects, magnets, and FB with complete obstruction demand emergent endoscopy. All other FBs with incomplete obstruction warrant urgent endoscopy [33].

The question whether to use flexible or rigid endoscopy greatly depends on the institutional policies. Flexible endoscopy is the first choice, as it is cost-effective and can be performed under sedation and local anesthesia. On the other hand, rigid endoscopy is superior for extraction of sharp objects and has the benefit of protected airways as it is always performed in general anesthesia [33, 34]. They are considered complementary techniques, equally effective for the removal of ingested FBs [35, 36].

Foley catheter can also be used for removal of FBs. It is used by inflating the balloon behind the FB and removing it with the extraction of the catheter. Although it has high success rate, it also has major disadvantages (no control of the FB and no airway control) [30, 37]. The use of this technique has been decreasing in recent years.

Esophageal bolus impaction can be treated by gently pushing it toward the stomach (90% success rate); however, extraction of the FB is preferred [33].

Surgical extraction of FB is usually reserved for irretrievable FBs and ones with complications such as perforation of the esophagus, fistula, extensive bleeding, and mediastinitis [33]. This is often a multidisciplinary endeavor and can be performed only in institutions of higher rang.

If the recurrent or unusual FB ingestion is observed, a mental health professional should be involved.

8. Inhaled foreign bodies

Foreign body aspiration is potentially one of the most urgent and the most stressful situations that can happen in a physician's career. Even a patient that presents as asymptomatic can quickly find itself in a life-threatening situation.

It occurs more often in children, particularly younger than 3 years of age [11, 38, 39], and is one of the leading causes of accidental death in this population [7]. Foreign body aspiration is less common in adults [40]. Risk factors in adult population include older age, neurological and mental disorders, alcoholism, sedative abuse, and tracheostomy cannula handling [39–41]. In most cases, aspiration happens accidentally; however, iatrogenic aspirations are also possible.

Inhaled FB are typically classified as organic or inorganic, with organic being the ones causing more complications. The most common organic FBs are bones and seeds, and the most common inorganic FBs are teeth, metallic and plastic objects [39, 40]. Teeth are one of the most prevalent iatrogenic FBs that can get broken off and displaced into the tracheobronchial tree during intubation or several ENT procedures [38].

FBs can be found in any part of tracheobronchial tree. Right bronchial tree is more often the place where FBs end up, due to its size and angle to the trachea. Lodgement in the trachea and especially larynx is far less common [42]. Localization of the FB greatly affects clinical presentation.

Symptoms range from acute respiratory distress to asymptomatic patients that do not even recall having aspirated an FB [38]. Cough is the most commonly occurring symptom, as it is a natural protective reflex of the body. Other common symptoms are dyspnea, stridor, wheezing, choking, hemoptysis, and chest pain [38]. Complications arise when the FB gets undetected for a longer period. Some of the possible complications are pneumonia, bronchiectasis, emphysema, empyema, and so forth. For that reason, in every patient with recurrent or long-standing pneumonia, FB must be considered [43, 44].

Detailed anamnesis and physical examination are in order. It is important to notice that ability to speak, cough, or breathe usually indicates that the patient has mild obstruction, while weakening of these parameters implies a severe airway obstruction [41]. If a conscious patient has a severe obstruction, back blows, abdominal, and chest thrusts can be of help. Efficacy of these measures increases if the patient is placed in a prone or a head-down position [45]. These treatments should not be used if the obstruction is mild since they can worsen the obstruction. If the patient is unresponsive, CPR should be started promptly [41].

In stable patients, posteroanterior and lateral chest radiographs are to be obtained when there is a suspicion of FB aspiration (**Figure A2**). However, not all FB can be seen on the radiograph; only 26% can be identified. Besides direct visualization, physician should be on the lookout for indirect radiograph findings of the FB, such as consolidation, atelectasis, air trapping, and mediastinal shift. It is important to note that normal radiograph finding does not exclude FB aspiration [39, 46]. CT scans are superior in detecting FB aspiration and providing information about the surrounding tissue, but they are not considered as a routine procedure for FB detection [46].

Bronchoscopy is a mainstay for treatment of inhaled FBs. Rigid bronchoscopy was first introduced by Gustav Killian in 1897 [47] and since then was used for FB extraction. With the improvement of flexible endoscopes, flexible bronchoscopy has become the standard tool in FB aspiration management [38]. Rigid bronchoscopy is usually preferred in children, while flexible bronchoscopy is considered as the first choice in adults, where it accounts for about 80–90% of retrieved FBs [39, 40]. As mentioned, when discussing ingested FBs, flexible and rigid endoscopies are considered complementary. The same applies for bronchoscopies. Flexible bronchoscopy provides better visualization, can be performed in the setting of local anesthesia and sedation, and is cheaper and faster to perform. On the other hand, rigid bronchoscopy provides better ventilation, has wide array of instruments that can be used during the extraction of FB, and is necessary in some cases (impacted, sharp, or large foreign bodies; cases with extensive granulation tissue or scaring; and several failed attempts of FB removal with flexible endoscopy) [38, 40].

When bronchoscopy fails to retrieve the FB, open surgery procedures may be necessary. It is particularly important in cases with recurrent complications. In some cases, tracheostomy needs to be performed to establish airway control. There have been a few cases in literature, where tracheostomy was performed to extract the FB since it was too big to pass through subglottis [48].

Complications of the extraction of inhaled FB include bleeding, trauma, asphyxiation, and so on. Granulation tissue often accompanies late-diagnosed FBs. Damage to this tissue leads to bleeding that is usually easily managed with cauterization. Trauma can occur at any part of the airway path during the management of the FB and may be the cause of later scaring. Even when the FB is secured by the instrument and extraction is in place, there is a danger of losing the grip and dropping the FB in the airway. If FB is big enough, it can get lodged into the trachea and cause a life-threatening situation. In this case, FB must be pushed into the distal parts of the airway to maintain partial ventilation. Once the ventilation is stabilized, attempt of extracting the FB must be repeated [38].

To his day, there are no valid clinical prediction models for FB aspiration. The decision relies on the astute clinical care tailored for each patient by an experienced clinician [49].

9. Special considerations

Button batteries, as an FB, are a medical emergency regardless of the localization. They are increasingly more present in every household device, such as toys, watches, remote controls, hearing aids, and so forth. Even though cylindrical batteries are also common FB, button batteries have significantly higher morbidity [27]. Because of their size and shape, button batteries get lodged in esophagus in such a way that both poles of the battery are touching the esophageal wall, establishing electrical current, which generates hydroxide radicals at the negative pole. Contrary to the assumption, thermal damage, pressure necrosis, and leakage of battery's internal substances (alkaline or lithium electrolytes) do not play a significant role in tissue damage [50–52]. Lithium batteries of ≥20 mm diameter pose the biggest risk. Damage to the mucosa of the esophageal wall occurs within 30 minutes and can be the cause of serious complications: esophageal perforation, tracheoesophageal fistula, aortoesophageal fistula, mediastinitis, and so on. This FB gives a characteristic finding on plain radiograph, similar to a coin, but with additional double halo rims. Button batteries are a clear indication for emergent endoscopic extraction [27, 34]. The application of oral honey (10 ml every 10 min) prior to extraction has recently been proposed by the National Capital Poison Center in the USA and in an ESPGHAN position paper in Europe, particularly for esophageal foreign bodies. Honey should be avoided in infants [52, 53]. After extraction, endoscopy should be repeated to assess the condition of esophagus and determine the risk for potential complications. Damage to the tissue may continue even after the extraction of the buttery if the site is not irrigated and environment neutralized. *Ex vivo* studies suggest that irrigating with mildly acidic beverages, such as lemon juice and soda or 50–150 mL of 0.25% sterile acetic acid, as early and frequently as possible may be most beneficial for pH neutralization [50, 52]. After removal of the button battery, patients should be on NPO (nil per os) and on careful observation since the above mentioned complications can happen several weeks after the FB removal. MRI is an important prognostic tool during this period [54].

The number of magnetic FB has been rising in the recent years. There is an increasing number of strong magnets (neodymium) in everyday objects. The attracting force of these magnets is many times stronger than that of conventional ones. When two magnets or a magnet and a metal object are ingested, they attract each other through the intestinal walls and can cause ischemia and tissue necrosis and consequentially obstruction, ulceration, perforation, fistulae, peritonitis, sepsis, and death. Symptoms depend on the size and the localization of the FBs. Patient may be asymptomatic or have abdominal pain and vomiting as the most common symptoms. Abdominal radiograph is essential for early diagnosis. Magnetic FB must be addressed promptly because every delay increases the risk of complications. Treatment is by endoscopic or surgical removal. If there is only one FB, observation may be considered with daily abdominal radiographs [25, 55].

Key points

- FB incidents are common and more prevalent in children.
- High level of suspicion is essential for FB diagnosis.
- Normal physical exam does not exclude FB diagnosis.

- Frontal and lateral plain radiographs are helpful, but normal findings do not exclude FB diagnosis.
- Button battery FB requires urgent removal.
- The majority of ingested FB are low-risk objects and pass through gastrointestinal tract without causing any problems.
- Bronchoscopy should be performed whenever there is a reasonable suspicion of aspirated FB.
- Recurrent or long-standing pulmonary problems warrant FB consideration.

Appendix

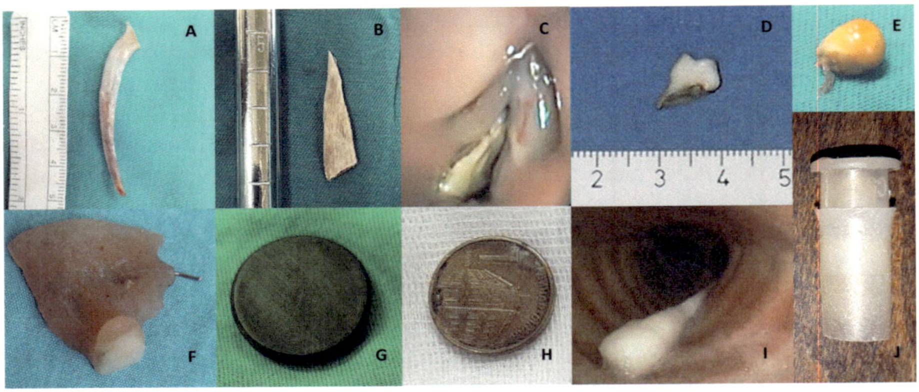

Figure A1.
Organic foreign bodies (A-E): A – bone form oesophagus; B – lamb bone from oesophagus; C – seed in glottis; D – tooth from right bronchus; E – corn from right bronchus. Inorganic foreign bodies (F-J): F – denture from oesophagus; G – magnet from oesophagus; H – coin from oesophagus; I – Q-tip in trachea; J – mouthpiece from left bronchus.

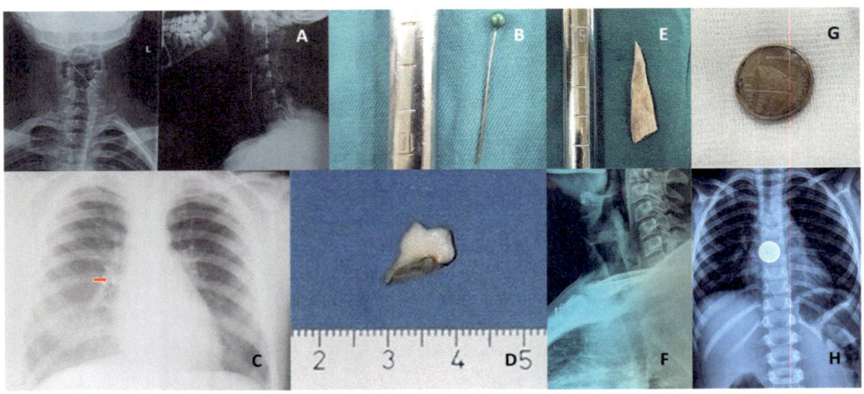

Figure A2.
Radiographs and extracted foreign bodies. A-B: needle in oesophagus; C-D: Tooth in right bronchus; E-F: lamb bone in oesophagus; G-H: oin in esophagus.

Author details

Dusan Milisavljevic[1,2*], Milan Stankovic[1,2], Nikola Djordjevic[1,2], Toma Kovacevic[1,2], Sasa Zivaljevic[2], Dragan Stojanov[2], Bojan Marinkovic[2] and Natalija Milisavljevic[1]

1 Faculty of Medicine, University of Niš, Niš, Serbia

2 ENT Clinic, University Clinical Centre Niš, Niš, Serbia

*Address all correspondence to: dusanorldusan@gmail.com

References

[1] Özcan K et al. Self-inserted foreign body and attention-deficit/hyperactivity disorder: Evaluated by the Conners' parent rating scales-revised. International Journal of Pediatric Otorhinolaryngology. 2013;**77**(12):1992-1997

[2] Mathew RP et al. Clinical presentation, diagnosis and management of aerodigestive tract foreign bodies in the adult population: Part 1. South African Journal of Radiology. 2021;**25**(1):2022

[3] Chen T et al. Pediatric esophageal foreign bodies: The role of socioeconomic status in ingestion patterns. Laryngoscope. Published online January 10, 2024. DOI: 10.1002/lary.31274

[4] El Khoury P et al. CT scan in children suspected of foreign body aspiration: A systematic review and meta-analysis. Otolaryngology and Head and Neck Surgery. 2024;**170**(1):1-12

[5] Panchabhai TS, Mehta AC. Historical perspectives of bronchoscopy. Connecting the dots. Annals of the American Thoracic Society. 2015;**12**(5):631-641

[6] Ho GC et al. A change in clinical practice for aural foreign bodies - what we learnt from the coronavirus disease 2019 pandemic. The Journal of Laryngology and Otology. 2021;**135**(9):825-828

[7] Brkic F et al. Death as a consequence of foreign body aspiration in children. Medical Archives. 2018;**72**(3):220-223

[8] Presentation of Data Frequencies on Foreign Body Injuries Cases in Children. The Susy Safe Registry as of March 6th 2023. Data Required Directly from the Susy Safe Registry. Available from: www.susysafe.org

[9] Aksakal C. Management of foreign bodies in the ear, nose and throat in children: A review of 829 cases from northern Anatolia. Otolaryngologia Polska. 2020;**74**(5):1-5

[10] Susy Safe Working Group. The Susy safe project overview after the first four years of activity. International Journal of Pediatric Otorhinolaryngology. 2012;**76**(Suppl. 1):S3-S11

[11] Salih AM, Alfaki M, Alam-Elhuda DM. Airway foreign bodies: A critical review for a common pediatric emergency. World Journal of Emergency Medicine. 2016;**7**(1):5-12

[12] Chiun KC et al. Review of ear, nose and throat foreign bodies in Sarawak general hospital. A five year experience. The Medical Journal of Malaysia. 2012;**67**(1):17-20

[13] Mingo K et al. Pediatric ear foreign body retrieval: A comparison across specialties. American Journal of Otolaryngology. 2020;**41**(2):102167

[14] White AC et al. Comparison of care settings for pediatric external auditory canal foreign bodies: A meta-analysis. The Annals of Otology, Rhinology, and Laryngology. 2023;**132**(3):322-331

[15] Weksler CW, Heiman E, Weiser G. Removal of external auditory canal foreign bodies in the pediatric emergency department - a retrospective comparison study. International Journal of Pediatric Otorhinolaryngology. 2022;**160**:111247

[16] Shih M, Brock L, Liu YC. Pediatric aural foreign body extraction:

Comparison of efficacies among clinical settings and retrieval methods. Otolaryngology and Head and Neck Surgery. 2021;**164**(3):662-666

[17] Grigg S, Grigg C. Removal of ear, nose and throat foreign bodies: A review. Australian Journal of General Practice. 2018;**47**(10):682-685

[18] Hira İ et al. Childhood nasal foreign bodies: Analysis of 1724 cases. Turkish Archives Of Otorhinolaryngology. 2019;**57**(4):187-190

[19] Jungbauer WN Jr et al. Comparison of pediatric nasal foreign body removal by care setting: A systematic review and meta-analysis. International Journal of Pediatric Otorhinolaryngology. 2022;**158**:111162

[20] Bance RRR et al. To X-ray or not to X-ray? Discussing unknown nasal foreign bodies and button batteries. Ear, Nose, & Throat Journal. 2024;**103**(1):Np49-np52

[21] Lee CH et al. Ear, nose, and throat foreign bodies in adults: A population-based study in Taiwan. Journal of the Formosan Medical Association. 2019;**118**(9):1290-1298

[22] Chen H et al. Migratory pharyngeal foreign bodies and related complications: Analysis of 20 cases. American Journal of Otolaryngology. 2022;**43**(2):103390

[23] Sueyoshi K et al. Fish bone descending in the mediastinum. Annals of Thoracic and Cardiovascular Surgery. 2023;**29**(6):323-325

[24] Birk M et al. Removal of foreign bodies in the upper gastrointestinal tract in adults: European Society of Gastrointestinal Endoscopy (ESGE) clinical guideline. Endoscopy. 2016;**48**(5):489-496

[25] Sutherland J, Bowen L. Ingestion of foreign bodies and caustic substances in children. BJA Education. 2023;**23**(1):2-7

[26] Gummin DD et al. 2022 annual report of the National Poison Data System(®) (NPDS) from America's poison centers(®): 40th annual report. Clinical Toxicology (Philadelphia, Pa.). 2023;**61**(10):717-939

[27] Kurowski JA, Kay M. Caustic ingestions and foreign bodies ingestions in pediatric patients. Pediatric Clinics of North America. 2017;**64**(3):507-524

[28] Evans DC et al. Intentional ingestions of foreign objects among prisoners: A review. World Journal of Gastrointestinal Endoscopy. 2015;**7**(3):162-168

[29] Destro F et al. Foreign body ingestion in neurologically impaired children: A challenging diagnosis and management in pediatric surgery. Children. 2021;**8**(11):956

[30] Dorterler ME, Günendi T. Foreign body and caustic substance ingestion in childhood. Open Access Emergency Medicine. 2020;**12**:341-352

[31] Yang TW et al. Diagnostic performance of conventional X-ray for detecting foreign bodies in the upper digestive tract: A systematic review and diagnostic meta-analysis. Diagnostics (Basel). 2021;**11**(5):790

[32] Klein A et al. Fish bone foreign body: The role of imaging. International Archives of Otorhinolaryngology. 2019;**23**(1):110-115

[33] Chirica M et al. Esophageal emergencies: WSES guidelines. World Journal of Emergency Surgery: WJES. 2019;**14**:26

[34] Demiroren K. Management of gastrointestinal foreign bodies with

brief review of the guidelines. Pediatric Gastroenterology, Hepatology & Nutrition. 2023;**26**(1):1-14

[35] Ferrari D et al. Flexible versus rigid endoscopy in the management of esophageal foreign body impaction: Systematic review and meta-analysis. World Journal of Emergency Surgery: WJES. 2018;**13**:42

[36] Tseng CC, Hsiao TY, Hsu WC. Comparison of rigid and flexible endoscopy for removing esophageal foreign bodies in an emergency. Journal of the Formosan Medical Association. 2016;**115**(8):639-644

[37] Choe JY, Choe BH. Foreign body removal in children using Foley catheter or magnet tube from gastrointestinal tract. Pediatric Gastroenterology, Hepatology & Nutrition. 2019;**22**(2): 132-141

[38] Bajaj D, Sachdeva A, Deepak D. Foreign body aspiration. Journal of Thoracic Disease. 2021;**13**(8):5159-5175

[39] Blanco Ramos M et al. Update in the extraction of airway foreign bodies in adults. Journal of Thoracic Disease. 2016;**8**(11):3452-3456

[40] Sehgal IS et al. Foreign body inhalation in the adult population: Experience of 25,998 bronchoscopies and systematic review of the literature. Respiratory Care. 2015;**60**(10):1438-1448

[41] Perkins GD et al. European resuscitation council guidelines for resuscitation 2015: Section 2. Adult basic life support and automated external defibrillation. Resuscitation. 2015;**95**:81-99

[42] Jain S et al. Impacted laryngeal foreign body in a child: A diagnostic and therapeutic challenge. Annals of Medical and Health Sciences Research. 2013;**3**(3):464-466

[43] Pritt B et al. A tale of three aspirations: Foreign bodies in the airway. Journal of Clinical Pathology. 2003;**56**(10):791-794

[44] Palasamudram Shekar S et al. Case of missing plastic: Foreign body bronchiectasis. Cureus. 2018;**10**(7):e2974

[45] Luczak A. Effect of body position on relieve of foreign body from the airway. AIMS Public Health. 2019;**6**(2):154-159

[46] Grassi R et al. Application of imaging guidelines in patients with foreign body ingestion or inhalation: Literature review. Seminars in Ultrasound, CT, and MR. 2015;**36**(1):48-56

[47] Killian G. Meeting of the Society of Physicians of Freiburg Dec 17, 1897. Münchener Medizinische Wochenschrift. 1898;**45**:378

[48] Fraga JC et al. Bronchoscopic removal of foreign body from airway through tracheotomy or tracheostomy. Jornal de Pediatria. 2003;**79**(4):369-372

[49] Lee JJW et al. Clinical prediction models for suspected pediatric foreign body aspiration: A systematic review and meta-analysis. JAMA Otolaryngology. Head & Neck Surgery. 2021;**147**(9):787-796

[50] Jatana KR, Barron CL, Jacobs IN. Initial clinical application of tissue pH neutralization after esophageal button battery removal in children. Laryngoscope. 2019;**129**(8):1772-1776

[51] Jatana KR et al. Basic mechanism of button battery ingestion injuries and novel mitigation strategies after diagnosis and removal. Laryngoscope. 2017;**127**(6):1276-1282

[52] Sethia R et al. Current management of button battery injuries. Laryngoscope Investigative Otolaryngology. 2021;**6**(3):549-563

[53] Schmidt YM, Muensterer O, Wendling-Keim D. The use of honey in button battery ingestions: A systematic review. Frontiers in Pediatrics. 2023;**11**:1259780

[54] Leinwand K, Brumbaugh DE, Kramer RE. Button battery ingestion in children: A paradigm for management of severe pediatric foreign body ingestions. Gastrointestinal Endoscopy Clinics of North America. 2016;**26**(1):99-118

[55] Altokhais T. Magnet ingestion in children management guidelines and prevention. Frontiers in Pediatrics. 2021;**9**:727988

Chapter 2

Foreign Bodies in ENT in Pediatric Age Group

Sameeksha Mishra and Sudhakar Vaidya

Abstract

The presence of foreign bodies (FB) in the ear, nose, and pharynx is indeed a common situation encountered by emergency physicians and otolaryngologists. These cases can pose significant challenges and, if not managed appropriately, may lead to life-threatening complications. It is crucial to promptly and carefully address these cases to prevent complications and ensure patient safety. As per day-to-day encountered cases, it was found that among the cases of foreign bodies (FBs) in pediatric patients presenting to the pediatric emergency unit, ear (otic) FBs accounted for the majority, nose (nasal) FBs were the second most common, and throat (pharyngolaryngeal) FBs were less frequent, the protocol for the removal of foreign bodies from the ear. It is crucial to have a systematic approach to ensure the safe and effective extraction of foreign bodies, especially in pediatric patients. This high occurrence can be attributed to the ease of identification and patient reporting, particularly for foreign bodies in accessible areas such as the ears, nose, and oropharynx. Overall, managing ear, nose, and throat (ENT) foreign bodies requires careful assessment, prompt intervention, and consideration of patient-specific factors to achieve successful outcomes while minimizing risks.

Keywords: foreign body, aerodigestive tract, esophagoscopy, button battery, cricopharynx

1. Introduction

The presence of foreign bodies (FB) in the ear, nose, and pharynx is indeed a common situation encountered by emergency physicians and otolaryngologists. These cases can pose significant challenges and, if not managed appropriately, may lead to life-threatening complications. It is crucial to promptly and carefully address these cases to prevent complications and ensure patient safety.

The statistics indicate that FB in the ear, nose, and pharynx collectively constitute a substantial proportion, accounting for 11% of all ENT emergencies. This highlights the importance of being well-prepared to handle such incidents in emergency settings.

The potential for life-threatening complications underscores the urgency of proper and timely management. Complications may include infections, perforations, or damage to surrounding structures. In the case of an ear, for example, a foreign body might damage the tympanic membrane or lead to infection in the ear canal.

In the nose or pharynx, complications may involve respiratory distress or damage to the airway. Medical professionals dealing with ENT emergencies need to stay updated on the latest protocols and techniques for managing foreign bodies. This includes having access to appropriate tools and equipment for safe removal and taking into consideration any specific challenges or risks associated with each case.

As per several studies and data from many studies regarding pediatric patients who presented to a pediatric emergency unit with foreign bodies in various anatomical locations such as the ear, nose, mouth/pharynx/tonsil, esophagus, and laryngotracheobronchial tree.

The following are analyzed:

1. *Demographic characteristics*: Age, gender, accompanying clinical findings.

2. *Foreign bodies (FBs)*: Localizations and types of FBs.

3. *Age analysis*: Evaluation of FB localizations by months.

4. *Physician expertise*: Evaluation of the expertise of physicians who removed FBs (emergency department physician, ENT specialist, pediatric surgeon, or chest surgeon).

5. *Methods of removal*: Evaluation of the methods used to remove FBs, categorized by anatomical regions and whether removal was performed with or without general anesthesia.

This is crucial for understanding the epidemiology, clinical presentation, and management strategies of foreign body ingestion or insertion in pediatric patients, which can help improve patient care and outcomes [1].

2. Pediatric pre ponderence

The observation that foreign bodies (FBs) in the ear, nose, and throat (ENT) cases are more prevalent in children under five years of age is consistent with existing literature. This age group is known for their curiosity, exploration of their surroundings, and lack of understanding of potential dangers, which can lead to the accidental insertion of foreign objects into various body orifices.

Several factors have been identified as contributing to the occurrence of FBs in this age group:

1. *Curiosity and exploration:* Young children are naturally curious and may insert objects into their ears, nose, or mouth to explore their body and surroundings.

2. *Boredom and games:* Children, when bored, may resort to playing with objects, and this can sometimes lead to the accidental insertion of items into their ears or nose.

3. *Intellectual disability and mental retardation:* Children with intellectual disabilities or mental retardation may have challenges understanding the consequences of their actions, making them more prone to inserting foreign bodies.

4. *Hyperactivity or attention deficit disorders:* Conditions such as hyperactivity or attention deficit disorders can contribute to impulsive behavior, increasing the likelihood of accidental insertion of foreign objects.

5. *Lack of careful caregivers:* Inadequate supervision or lack of attentive caregivers can also play a role in children accessing objects that may pose a risk.

The diversity of foreign bodies may vary based on anatomical regions, indicating that the choice of objects and the methods of insertion may differ. For example, objects lodged in the ear may differ from those in the nose or throat due to the specific anatomical features and accessibility of each region.

3. Sites of FB

As per day-to-day encountered cases, it was found that among the cases of foreign bodies (FBs) in pediatric patients presenting to the pediatric emergency unit:

- ear (otic) FBs accounted for the majority,
- nose (nasal) FBs were the second most common, and
- throat (pharyngolaryngeal) FBs were less frequent,

This breakdown provides valuable insight into the distribution of FBs among different anatomical locations, which can help guide clinical management protocols and resource allocation in the pediatric emergency setting.

Most common foreign bodies in practice:

Based on the data:

- Seeds (corns/beans/rice husk/wheat) are the most common foreign bodies removed from the ear, nose, and throat.
- Among these, 42 cases (17.6%) were found in children.
- Cotton buds were another common foreign body also found in children aged 10 years and below.
- Beads constituted a significant portion of nasal and ear foreign bodies. Additionally, the majority of beads are found in children.

4. FB in aerodigestive tract

Frequency of foreign bodies aspirated or ingested, classified into inorganic and organic types. Here's a breakdown of the data presented (**Table 1**):

This table, taken from a valued study, provides a detailed breakdown of the types of foreign bodies aspirated or ingested, categorized by their classification as inorganic or organic. It also includes the frequency of each type and the percentage distribution of aspiration and ingestion within each classification (These cases were studied in

Classification	Type	Frequency	Total	Aspiration (%)	Ingestion (%)
Inorganic	Denture	20	20	100	0
	Metallic bolt/screw/cap	3	4	75	25
	Disc-lithium watch battery	4	4	100	0
	LED bulb	2	2	100	0
	Ear ring	2	2	100	0
	Biro base cork	2	2	100	0
	Office pin	2	2	100	0
	Plastic whistle/ball/doll valve	4	4	100	0
	Coin	1	1	100	0
	Plastic bead	1	1	100	0
	Sharpener	1	1	100	0
	Metallic washer	1	1	100	0
	Key	1	1	100	0
Organic	Kolanut	1	2	50	50
	Sugarcane peel	1	1	100	0
	Peanut	3	3	100	0
	Vegetable	1	1	100	0
	Maize	1	1	100	0
	Not stated	2	9	22.2	77.8
	No object seen	3	3	100	0
	Not applicable	0	1	0	100
	TOTAL	28	66	42.4	57.6

Table 1.
Types of foreign bodies with their frequency of aspiration and ingestion.

the said hospital of the stated reference shows different kind of foreign bodies in the same area, and these cases are more or less similar in all other region as well since the pediatric age group commonly involved).

The prevalence of these foreign bodies is almost similar all around as the pediatric preponderance is common as we have already read [2].

5. Removal of FB

The protocol for the removal of foreign bodies from the ear. It is crucial to have a systematic approach to ensure the safe and effective extraction of foreign bodies, especially in pediatric patients. Here is a summary of the steps:

1. *Outpatient Department (OPD) Removal*:

    - Foreign bodies that are easily removable through suction or manual extraction under vision (using a microscope, endoscope, or naked eye) can be managed in the OPD setting.

- This approach is suitable for cases where the foreign body is readily visible and accessible, and the patient can cooperate during the procedure.

2. *Operating room (OR) removal*:

- If the foreign body is not easily retractable or poses a risk of complications during removal, the procedure may need to be performed in the operating room under anesthesia.

- Anesthesia ensures the patient's comfort and cooperation, which is especially important for pediatric patients who may not tolerate invasive procedures well.

- Removal under anesthesia allows for a more controlled environment, reducing the risk of injury or further complications.

By following this protocol, healthcare providers can ensure the safe and efficient removal of foreign bodies from the ear, taking into account factors such as the nature of the foreign body, patient cooperation, and the need for anesthesia, particularly in pediatric cases.

The removal of foreign bodies from the nose:

1. *Outpatient department (OPD) removal:*

- Foreign bodies that are easily removable through suction or manual extraction under direct visualization can be managed in the OPD setting.

- This approach is suitable for cases where the foreign body is accessible and can be safely extracted without the need for anesthesia.

2. *Operating room (OR) removal*:

- In cases where the foreign body is not easily retrievable or poses a risk of complications during removal, such as in older cases, removal in the operating room under anesthesia is preferable.

- Anesthesia ensures patient comfort and cooperation, particularly in cases where the procedure may be more complex or uncomfortable.

- Removal under anesthesia allows for a controlled environment, reducing the risk of injury and ensuring thorough removal of the foreign body.

3. *Endoscopic guidance*:

- Endoscopic guidance can be beneficial, especially in cases involving maggots or complex foreign bodies that may require visualization beyond what is possible with naked-eye examination.

- Endoscopy provides a clear view of the nasal cavity, facilitating precise removal of the foreign body and ensuring thorough inspection for any additional complications, such as tissue damage or secondary infections.

By following these guidelines, healthcare providers can effectively manage foreign bodies in the nose, ensuring safe and thorough removal while minimizing discomfort and complications for the patient.

Exactly foreign bodies lodged in the throat or aerodigestive tract often require specialized techniques for safe and effective removal. Here are some common methods:

1. *Esophagoscopy:*
    - Esophagoscopy involves the insertion of a flexible or rigid endoscope through the mouth to visualize and remove foreign bodies lodged in the esophagus.
    - Flexible esophagoscopy is preferred for its ability to navigate through the curves of the esophagus, offering a less invasive and more comfortable option for the patient.
    - Rigid esophagoscopy may be necessary for certain cases where a more direct approach is required or when dealing with larger or more challenging foreign bodies.
2. *Laryngoscopy*:
    - Laryngoscopy is used to visualize and remove foreign bodies lodged in the larynx or upper part of the throat.
    - It can be performed using a flexible or rigid endoscope, depending on the specific location of the foreign body and the patient's condition.
    - Flexible laryngoscopy allows for a detailed examination of the larynx and surrounding structures with minimal discomfort to the patient.
    - Rigid laryngoscopy may be employed for cases requiring a more direct approach or when dealing with complex foreign bodies.
3. *Bronchoscopy:*

It is indeed a valuable and often essential procedure for the removal of aspirated foreign bodies from the bronchus. Here is why it is considered promising:

1. *Direct visualization*: Bronchoscopy allows physicians to directly visualize the bronchial tree, providing clear imaging of the foreign body's location and facilitating precise removal.
2. *Flexibility*: Bronchoscopes come in flexible and rigid forms, allowing healthcare providers to choose the most appropriate instrument based on the patient's anatomy and the nature of the foreign body.
3. *Minimally invasive*: Bronchoscopy is minimally invasive compared to traditional surgical methods for removing bronchial foreign bodies. It can often be performed under sedation or general anesthesia, depending on the patient's condition and the complexity of the procedure.

4. *Effective removal*: With bronchoscopy, foreign bodies can be safely and effectively removed from the bronchial tree, reducing the risk of complications such as pneumonia, lung collapse, or chronic inflammation.

5. *Diagnostic and therapeutic*: Bronchoscopy serves both diagnostic and therapeutic purposes. In addition to removing foreign bodies, it allows for the assessment of airway integrity and the identification of any associated injuries or abnormalities.

6. *Reduced complications*: Compared to alternative methods, bronchoscopy typically results in fewer complications and shorter recovery times for patients.

Overall, bronchoscopy plays a crucial role in the management of aspirated foreign bodies in the bronchus, offering a safe, effective, and minimally invasive approach to diagnosis and treatment.

Both esophagoscopy and laryngoscopy are valuable tools in the removal of foreign bodies from the throat or aerodigestive tract, providing healthcare providers with the ability to safely visualize and extract the foreign body while minimizing the risk of complications. The choice between flexible and rigid techniques depends on factors such as the nature of the foreign body, the patient's anatomy, and the expertise of the medical team.

6. Complications of FB removal

While the removal of foreign bodies (FBs) from various anatomical sites such as the ear, nose, throat, and bronchus is generally safe, certain complications can occur, particularly if the procedure is not performed carefully or if the FB is lodged deeply or in a delicate area. Some potential complications include:

1. *Perforation*: Perforation refers to the unintended puncturing of tissue or organs during the removal procedure. This can occur if excessive force is applied or if the FB is sharp and causes damage to surrounding structures. Perforation can lead to further complications such as infection, bleeding, or organ dysfunction.

2. *Bleeding*: Bleeding can occur during or after FB removal, especially if the FB has caused trauma to blood vessels or delicate mucosal tissues. Factors such as the size and location of the FB, the patient's underlying health conditions, and the technique used for removal can influence the risk of bleeding.

3. *Infection*: Infection may occur if the FB or the removal procedure introduces bacteria into the affected area. This risk is particularly high in cases where the FB has been present for an extended period or if multiple attempts at removal are made.

4. *Airway compromise*: In cases of FB removal from the upper airway (such as the nose, throat, or bronchus), there is a risk of airway compromise if the FB becomes dislodged and obstructs the airway. This can lead to respiratory distress or even respiratory arrest if not promptly managed.

5. *Damage to surrounding structures*: Depending on the location of the FB and the technique used for removal, there is a risk of damage to surrounding structures such as nerves, blood vessels, or adjacent organs. This can result in pain, sensory deficits, or functional impairment.

6. *Aspiration*: During FB removal, there is a risk of the FB being accidentally aspirated into the lower airway, especially if the patient coughs or moves suddenly. Aspiration can lead to respiratory complications such as pneumonia or lung abscess.

To minimize the risk of complications during FB removal, healthcare providers must carefully assess each case, choose appropriate techniques and instruments, and ensure proper patient monitoring and follow-up care. In cases where complications occur, prompt recognition and intervention are essential to prevent further harm and facilitate optimal recovery.

6.1 Different types of FB removal

See (**Figures 1–6**).

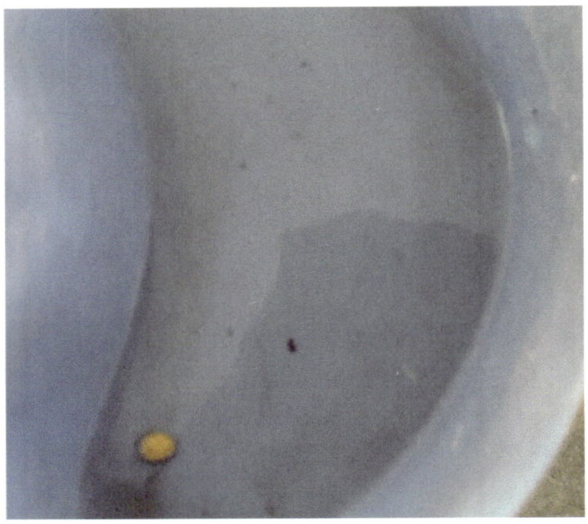

Figure 1.
A soybean removed from ear.

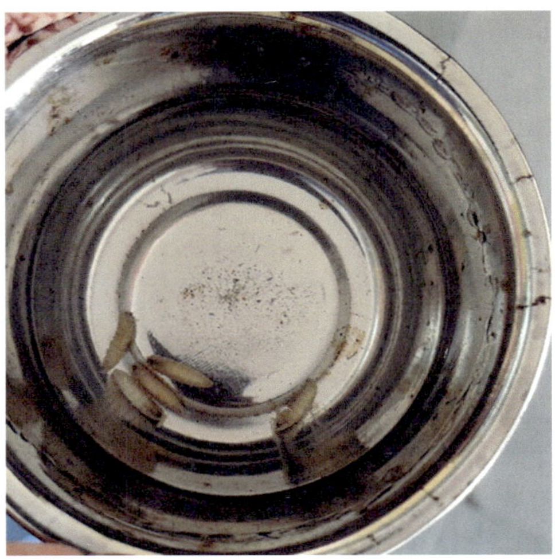

Figure 2.
Maggots removed from nasal cavity.

DOI: http://dx.doi.org/10.5772/intechopen.1005815

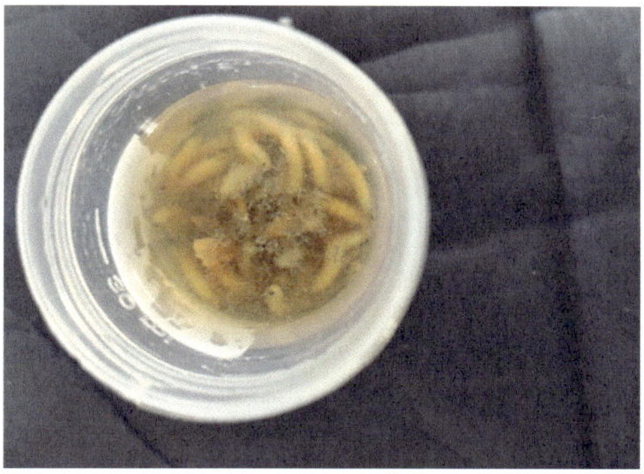

Figure 3.
Maggots.

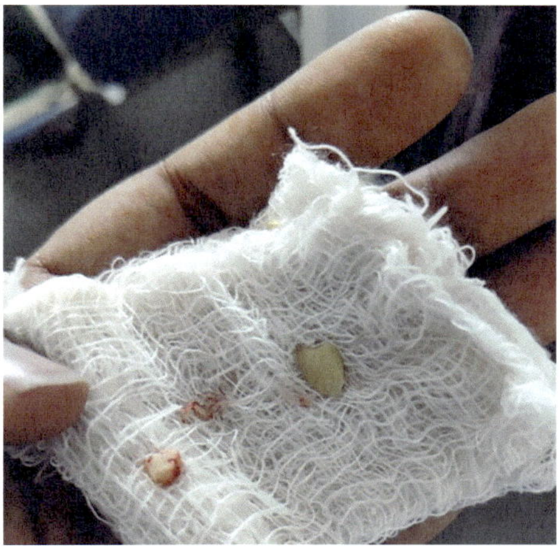

Figure 4.
Broken pieces of bean from ear.

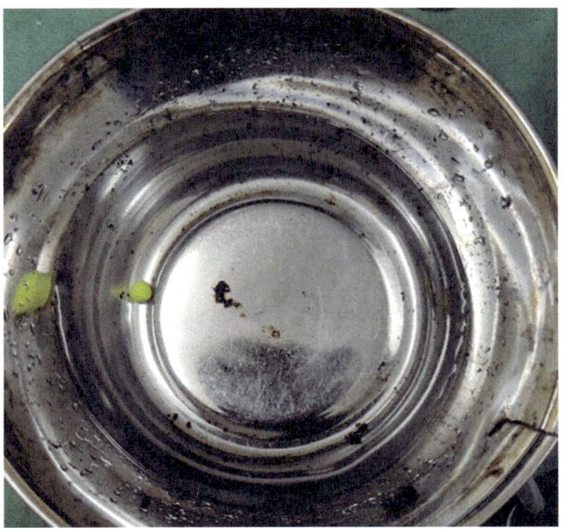

Figure 5.
Yellow pearl from ear.

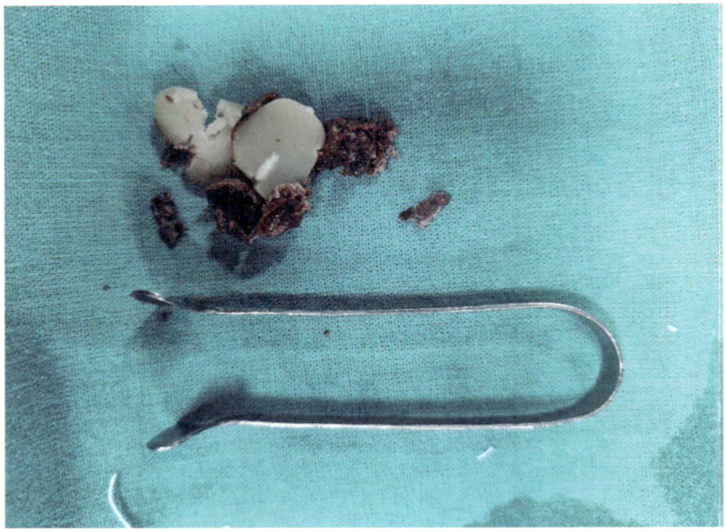

Figure 6.
Broken grain pieces from nasal cavity.

7. Discussion

The prevalence of ENT (ear, nose, and throat) foreign bodies reported by our center aligns with findings from other studies, indicating that ENT foreign bodies are a common issue in healthcare settings. This high occurrence can be attributed to the ease of identification and patient reporting, particularly for foreign bodies in accessible areas such as the ears, nose, and oropharynx.

Foreign bodies were most frequently found in the ears, followed by the nose and oropharynx, which is consistent with existing literature. Some studies have suggested a specific order of frequency and location for foreign bodies, including the ears, nose, pharynx, esophagus, and tracheobronchial tree.

Complementary tests are rarely required for diagnosing foreign bodies, as direct visualization during physical examination is usually sufficient. However, in some cases, complementary tests such as X-ray imaging may be necessary, particularly for identifying radio-opaque foreign bodies. It is important to note that X-ray imaging may not be effective for diagnosing radiolucent objects like fish and chicken bones.

The types of foreign bodies encountered can vary based on social and geographic factors. For example, developing countries may see more cases involving cotton seeds and fragments, while developed countries may encounter small plastic parts more frequently.

Prompt and atraumatic removal of foreign bodies is essential, but the success of removal depends on various factors, and no single method has been shown to be superior. However, leaving foreign bodies in ENT cavities for extended periods or repeated attempts at removal can increase the risk of complications and reduce the chances of success.

Overall, managing ENT foreign bodies requires careful assessment, prompt intervention, and consideration of patient-specific factors to achieve successful outcomes while minimizing risks [3]. One more study that we have taken as reference included 119 patients with ages ranging from 8 months to 13.83 years (median 3.67 years).

Forty-nine cases had a definite history of FBs ingestion, with a residence time varying from 10 h to 5 years. The rest of the 70 patients were identified under imaging examination or surgical exploration [4]. According to a recent study foreign bodies (FBs) in pediatric otorhinolaryngology represent up to 10% of cases in emergency departments (ED) and are primarily present in children under five years old. They are probably the result of children's curiosity and tendency to explore the environment [5].

Another good example of study which we have included is a hospital based cross-sectional retrospective study was performed in the Department of ENT and Head neck Surgery at Chandulal Chandrakar Memorial Medical College, Bhilai, Chhattisgarh, which is a tertiary referral teaching institute of central India. The study population included all patients presenting with lodgement of foreign bodies in ear, nose, throat, aerodigestive tract and maxillofacial region in the Outpatient Department (OPD) or in the emergency ward during the 4 year study period (from January 2015 to December 2018). Data was collected from ENT clinic registration books and ward admission records [6].

All these studies have helped us to frame the chapter structure.

8. Conclusion

Understanding these age-specific characteristics is crucial for healthcare providers when managing foreign body cases in pediatric patients. Prompt recognition and appropriate intervention are essential to prevent complications associated with aspiration, which can be more critical than cases involving ingestion. Aspiration of foreign bodies can lead to respiratory distress, pneumonia, and other severe respiratory complications.

Additionally, the recognition of a male preponderance in pediatric cases may guide preventive strategies and educational efforts targeting parents and caregivers, helping them create safer environments for young children. It emphasizes the importance of age-appropriate supervision and childproofing measures to minimize the risk of accidental ingestion or aspiration of foreign bodies during play.

In summary, the age-specific behaviors and physiological characteristics of young children contribute to their increased vulnerability to foreign body incidents, emphasizing the need for tailored approaches in both prevention and management in pediatric cases [7]. Ensuring children are safe from ingesting or inhaling small objects is a top priority. Parents and caregivers should be educated on the risks of small items that can block airways or cause choking. Remember, prevention is the best remedy to ensure children's safety [8].

Acknowledgements

The authors are thankful to the Managing Director of R.D. Gardi Medical College, Ujjain Dr. V.K. Mahadik, for his constant support and supervision.

I, Dr. Sameeksha Mishra, show my gratitude to my HOD and co-author in this chapter, Dr. Sudhakar Vaidya, Professor and HOD R.D. Gardi Medical College Ujjain, who has been the torch bearer to my academic work since the start of my career, I can never thank him enough. The author acknowledges the use of ChatGPT 4.0 for language polishing of the manuscript in several sentences, however most of the editing is done personally.

Conflict of interest

The authors declare no conflict of interest.

Acronyms and abbreviations

FB	foreign body
ENT	ear, nose, and throat
OR	operating room
OPD	outpatient department

Author details

Sameeksha Mishra[1*] and Sudhakar Vaidya[2]

1 Rama Medical College and Hospital, Ghaziabad, UP, India

2 R.D Gardi Medical College, Ujjain, MP, India

*Address all correspondence to: drsameeksha.06@gmail.com

References

[1] Aksakal C. Management of foreign bodies in the ear, nose and throat in children: A review of 829 cases from northern Anatolia. Otolaryngologia Polska. 2020;**74**(5):1-5. DOI: 10.5604/01.3001.0014.1579

[2] Adedeji TO, Sogebi OA, Bande S. Clinical spectrum of ear, nose and throat foreign bodies in North Western Nigeria. African Health Sciences. 2016;**16**(1): 292-297. DOI: 10.4314/ahs.v16i1.38

[3] Adeoye PO, Afolabi OA, Omokanye HK, Olaoye I, Akanbi OR, Segun-Busari S, et al. Foreign bodies in the aerodigestive tract: Time for comprehensive preventive measures. African Health Sciences. 2022;**22**(2): 369-376. DOI: 10.4314/ahs.v22i2.42

[4] Chen QJ, Wang LY, Chen Y, Xue JJ, Zhang YB, Zhang LF, et al. Management of foreign bodies ingestion in children. World Journal of Pediatrics. 2022;**18**(12):854-860. DOI: 10.1007/s12519-022-00585-7

[5] Paladin I, Mizdrak I, Gabelica M, Golec Parčina N, Mimica I, Batinović F. Foreign bodies in pediatric otorhinolaryngology: A review. Pediatric Reports. 2024;**16**(2):504-518. DOI: 10.3390/pediatric16020042

[6] Kekre M, Chakravarty S, Agarwal R. Foreign bodies in ear, nose, throat and maxillofacial region: A study on their clinical profile and complications. Indian Journal of Otolaryngology and Head & Neck Surgery. 2022;**74**(Suppl 3):4483-4494. DOI: 10.1007/s12070-020-02233-w

[7] Mangussi-Gomes J, Andrade JS, Matos RC, Kosugi EM, Penido NO. ENT foreign bodies: Profile of the cases seen at a tertiary hospital emergency care unit. Brazilian Journal of Otorhinolaryngology. 2013;**79**(6):699-703. DOI: 10.5935/1808-8694.20130128

[8] Ahmed ME, Refaie BM, Ahmed ME, Ali AHA, Dahy KG. Foreign body swallows with airway affection in pediatrics. Indian Journal of Otolaryngology and Head & Neck Surgery. 2023;**75**(2):287-291. DOI: 10.1007/s12070-022-03156-4

Chapter 3

Perspective Chapter: Classification and Complications of Aerodigestive Button Batteries and Magnets

Hardip Singh Gendeh and Balwant Singh Gendeh

Abstract

Aerodigestive foreign bodies is a term used to group together airway foreign bodies and oesophageal foreign bodies. Anatomically, the cricopharyngeus is the narrowest part of the airway among the paediatric population with high risks of airway foreign body impaction. Button batteries account for less than 2% of the foreign bodies ingested in children. Non-organic aerodigestive foreign body ingestion is common in children. Button batteries and magnets pose a serious risk of injury and complications. Majority are unwitnessed, requiring a high index of suspicion among children presenting with abdominal discomfort. Urgent removal is indicated.

Keywords: aerodigestive, foreign bodies, button batteries, magnets, classification, complications

1. Introduction

Aerodigestive foreign bodies is a term used to group together airway foreign bodies and oesophageal foreign bodies. This is because the airway and oesophagus are closely related, sharing the same pathway via the nasopharynx and oropharynx prior to going its separate routes to the oesophagus posteriorly and the trachea anteriorly. At the level of the oropharynx, the oesophagus is a continuation from the cricopharyngeus which is the narrowest part of the oesophagus forming the upper oesophageal sphincter. The cricopharynx consists of the cricopharyngeus muscle that undergoes concentric contraction as its motor function. The swallowing within the oesophagus undergoes three processes which are tonicity, relaxation, and peristalsis to propel food into the stomach and prevent reflux [1]. Anteriorly, the larynx is the gateway to the trachea inferiorly. Prior to reaching the trachea, the subglottic lies just inferior to the larynx, and it is bounded by the cricoid cartilage This possesses to be the narrowest part of an airway among the paediatric population, with high risks of airway foreign body impaction occurring here.

The objective of this chapter is to discuss the classification of aerodigestive foreign bodies and the complications associated with button battery and magnet aerodigestive injury. For this chapter, the authors utilised PubMed and Google Scholar using searches button battery. AND aerodigestive AND complications; and magnet AND aerodigestive AND complications. Relevant manuscripts or manuscripts with a different perspective were selected.

2. Classification

There are several ways to classify foreign bodies. They can be classified based on the anatomical structure in which they are trapped within. Aerodigestive foreign bodies can be classified into organic or inorganic foreign bodies [2]. This is the preference of the authors as their demographics, symptomatology, and management may be different. Organic foreign bodies are derived from natural substances and may consist of food. They are often radiolucent and are higher in the adult population. This is because a healthy adult is less likely to purposefully insert foreign bodies into the aerodigestive tract unless ingested with food. Inorganic foreign bodies are processed foreign bodies such as wood and metal objects. They are common in children as they are often purposefully inserted and are often radiopaque [2]. Less than one third of aerodigestive foreign bodies are radiopaque on a chest radiograph [3].

Up to 90% of foreign bodies that unintentionally inserted will pass through the aerodigestive tract are asymptomatic and cause no harm. They do not require any intervention. On the other hand, almost 80% of intentionally inserted foreign bodies require some form of intervention [4].

The term foreign body aspiration is used when a foreign body is aspirated into the airways or lungs. Ingestion on the other hand occurs when the foreign body is swallowed into the digestive tract [5]. Foreign body injury is the term used to describe the damage caused by the foreign body inhalation or aspiration to the organ [2]. Therefore, the authors prefer to use the term foreign body injury when dealing with its complications.

The complications caused by a foreign body injury depend on several factors, i.e. size, shape, and rigidity. Spherical objects and sharp objects are predominant with choking or perforation hazards, respectively [2, 6]. Complications are best described according to the anatomical structure, but a magnet and battery foreign bodies are highlighted and discussed in detail in this chapter.

3. Button battery foreign bodies

The recent development of technology has accelerated the broad use of button batteries. Button batteries are increasingly used in devices such as hearing aids, electronic games, watches, digitalised planners, and new electronic gadgets. Furthermore, it is readily available among electronic gadgets used by children or made accessible to them such as electronic toys and remote controls. Button battery foreign bodies may have a fatal outcome. Conversely, it may result in little to no ill effect on a child.

Button batteries although attractive to children due to their shape and shiny surface account for less than 2% of the total foreign bodies ingested among the paediatric population [7–10].

Smaller batteries are easily inserted into the orifices of the nose and ear instead of being aspirated or ingested. A study that reviewed button batteries among 13 children in a hospital in Egypt showed that it was present in the nose (5), oesophagus (4), stomach (3), and external auditory meatus (1) [11]. Conventional button batteries may leak as early as 2 hours once within the aerodigestive tract resulting in localised tissue damage [12].

3.1 Signs and symptoms

Children with button battery foreign bodies may present with variable symptoms. Some children may present with no signs or symptoms while others have non-specific signs like pain, cough, vomiting, irritability, fever, and tachycardia. More specific symptoms include drooling, dysphagia, nasal discharge, epistaxis, nasal blockage, breathing difficulty, vomiting, choking, and cough.

3.2 Complications

In the nose, the presence of bony projections from the lateral wall called turbinate hinders the insertion of button batteries beyond the nasal cavity causing the battery to be trapped within it. If it is lodged at the area between the turbinate and septum known as the meatus, the exposed surface area is larger. Complications for a nasal button battery include septal perforation, mucosal ulceration, and necrosis of the turbinate (**Figure 1**) [10]. Oesophageal button batteries may result in mucosal oedema, mucosal necrosis or burns, and perforation (**Figures 2–4**). This may lead to sepsis or mediastinitis. The similar may be the same for gastric button batteries although the Egyptian study had no complications with all three children having passed the button battery in the stool after several days. Erythema, oedema, and necrosis of the external

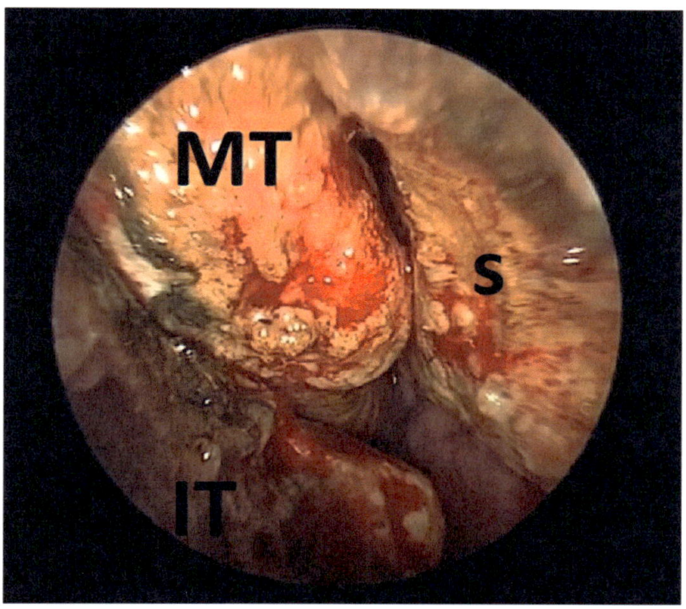

Figure 1.
Nasal endoscopy image after removal of a button battery. Necrosis (black areas) and unhealthy mucosa of the right nasal cavity. A button battery was lodged at the right inferior meatus for over 24 hours in a 4-year-old child. MT: middle turbinate; S: nasal septum; IT: inferior turbinate. Fortunately, the child did not develop a septal perforation.

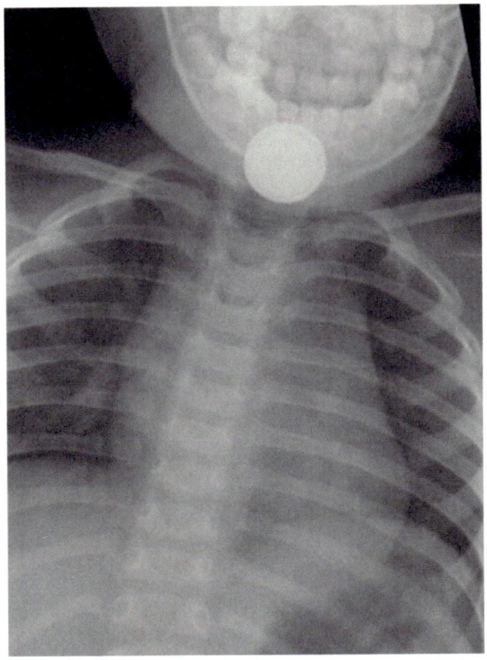

Figure 2.
AP radiograph of an oesophageal button battery.

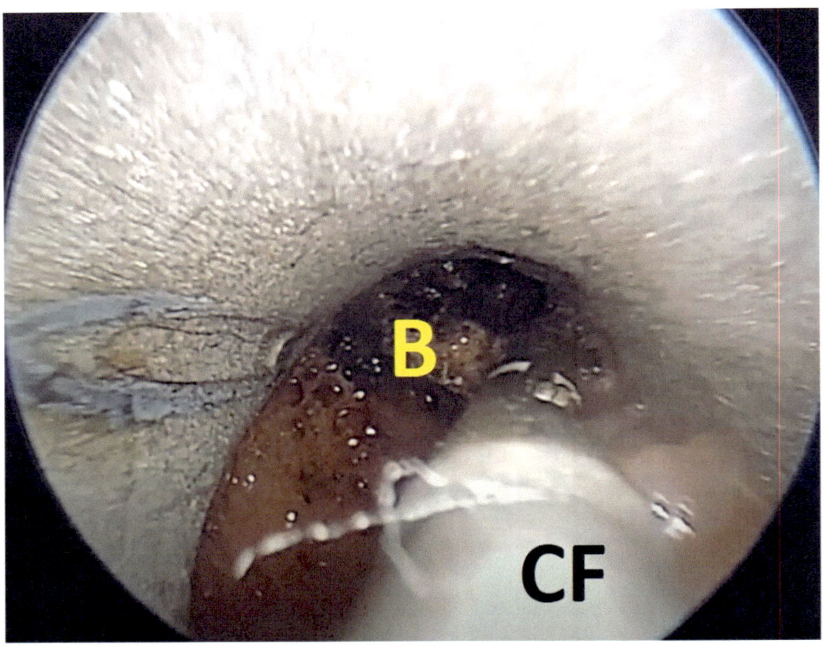

Figure 3.
Direct laryngoscopy view of removal of an oesophageal button battery (B) from the cricopharyngeus. The battery was adherent to the surrounding mucosa requiring force with a crocodile forceps (CF) to be released from the cricopharyngeus.

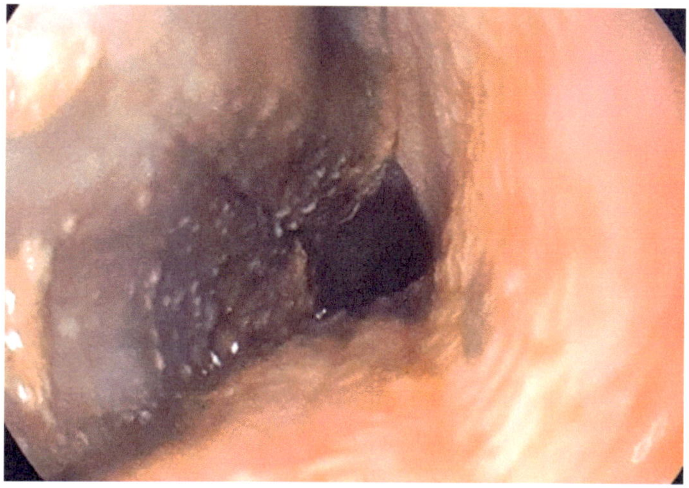

Figure 4.
Rigid oesophagoscopy showing oesophageal necrosis of the left oesophagus (blackish areas) post button battery removal.

ear canal may occur, and tympanic membrane perforation is possible when a button battery is inserted into the ear. Other complications are saddling nose due to a large area of septal cartilage perforation, septal chondritis, scarring resulting in atrophic rhinitis, and nasal mucosal synechiae or stenosis [13, 14].

Button batteries cause trauma to the surrounding mucosa via the following mechanisms.

1. The higher body temperature causes leakage of the corrosive battery contents resulting in local trauma or burns.

2. The button battery being a solid object being wedged within nasal mucosa may cause pressure necrosis.

3. Button batteries when exposed to the moist aerodigestive mucosa may cause the formation of eddy currents or small circuit of currents resulting in electrical burns and trauma to the exposed mucosa

4. Substance released may be absorbed by the mucosa resulting in delayed localised trauma and liquifying necrosis.

3.3 Investigations

Being inorganic and made of metal, button batteries are easily confirmed via its opacity within the radiograph. In unwitnessed ingestions, it may be confusing if the spherical radiopacity is a button battery or a coin. A halo sign which is a double rim at the peripherals of the sphere is present in a button battery in the anterior–posterior radiograph (**Figure 5**). In the lateral view, a step sign may help identify a button battery (**Figures 6** and 7). The positive pole forms the outer larger cap which fits over the smaller negative pole. The difference in diameter between the positive and negative pole gives rise to the halo sign and step sign [15]. This is a reliable predictor of a button battery.

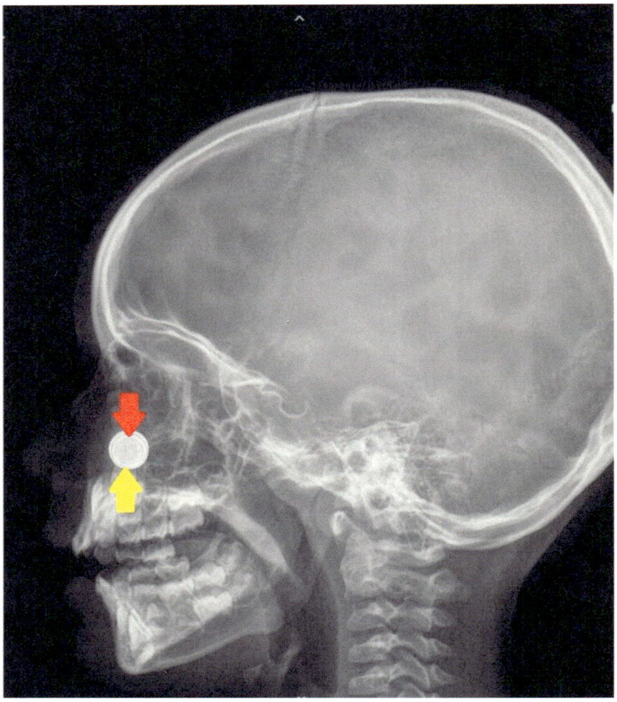

Figure 5.
Lateral radiograph view of the button battery in the patient in ***Figure 1****. The halo sign can be appreciated. The outer circle (red arrow) is formed by the larger positive cap while the inner circle (yellow arrow) is formed by the smaller negative cap.*

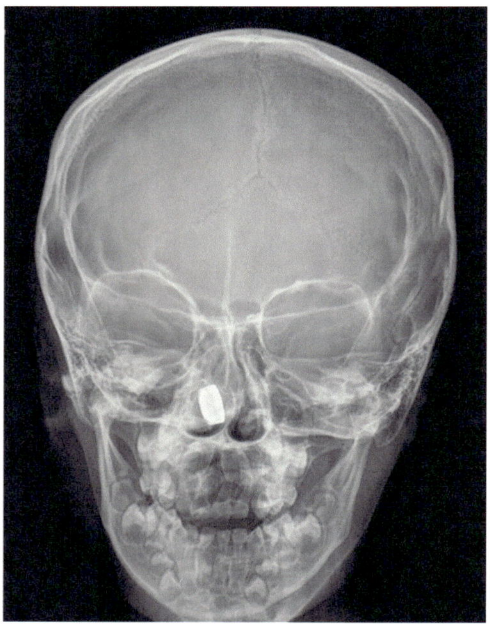

Figure 6.
AP radiograph view of the button battery in the patient in ***Figure 1*** *which is located in the inferior meatus.*

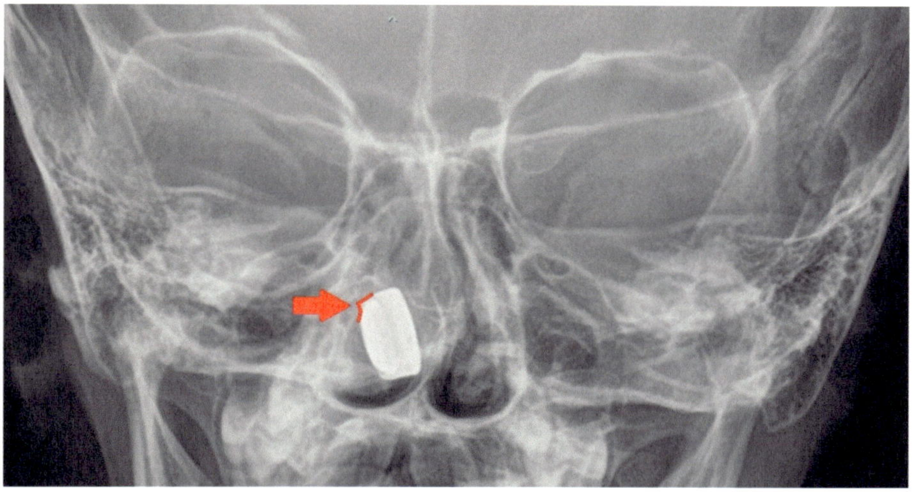

Figure 7.
*Magnification of **Figure 4** with the step sign seen in the AP view. In this radiograph, the button battery was at an angle resulting in a less clear step sign.*

However, the author has presented one case whereby the patient ingested two coins of varying diameter resulting in a pseudo halo sign and step sign as they were stacked side by side in the oesophagus. This, however, is a rare incident [15, 16].

3.4 Management

For nasal button batteries, urgent removal (preferably below 2–4 hours) is recommended to minimise local trauma to surrounding tissues. Most batteries can be removed under endoscopic guidance under general anaesthesia or local anaesthesia as the earlier is preferred if local trauma is suspected (**Figure 8**). Granulation tissues and necrotic tissues should be removed and debrided. The cavity should be rinsed with normal saline to wash away any chemical contaminants. Shall there be loss of septal mucosa or perforation, the authors prefer a silastic sheath which may be kept in for 2 weeks to act as a scaffolding for re-epithelialisation of the septum and prevention of synechiae (**Figure 9**). A silastic sheath may be difficult to remove in an uncooperative child, and a second procedure under general anaesthesia can be planned for re-assessment, toileting, and removal of silastic sheath. Shall there be a permanent septal perforation, it should be treated clinically. Septal perforations can be managed conservatively if they are asymptomatic, consideration of septal button if they are small and surgical management if it is symptomatic and large.

Similar to oesophageal button batteries, an oesophageal-gastro-duodenoscopy (OGDS) or rigid oesophagoscopy can be performed. If perforation is suspected, a nasogastric tube should be inserted under endoscopic guidance to rest the oesophagus. Broad-spectrum antibiotics can be started, and a post-operative chest radiograph should be performed. One should watch out for mediastinitis. Most oesophageal perforations heal within 2 weeks. A barium swallow can be performed prior to recommencing oral feeds.

Shall the button battery have passed the oesophagus into the stomach; the guidelines recommend observational with serial radiographs up to 2 weeks. Endoscopic removal should be considered if the battery has not passed through the stomach.

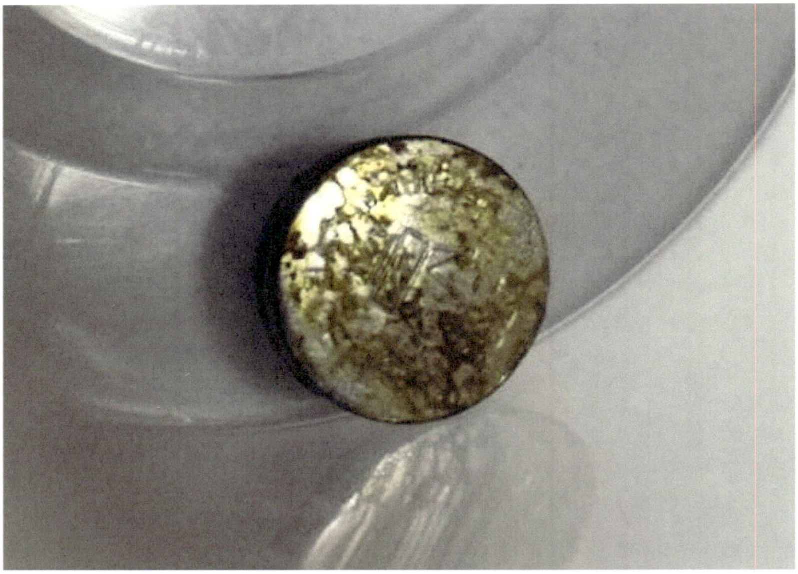

Figure 8.
Button battery removed via endoscopic guidance after 24 hours. Note the discoloration on the battery caused by chemical release and electrical burns of the mucosa.

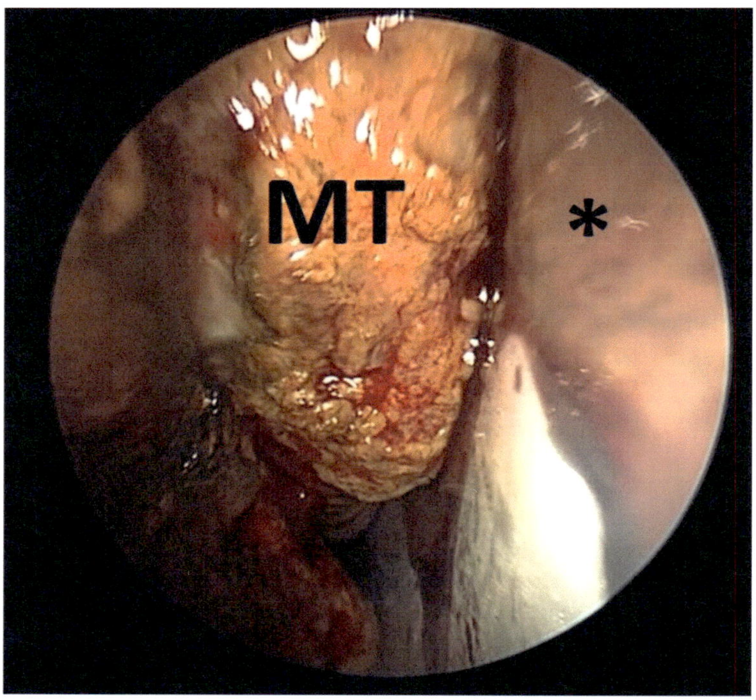

Figure 9.
*Silastic sheath (labelled *) inserted between the septum and the middle turbinate (MT) allows for re-epithelialisation of the nasal septal mucosa and prevents adhesion between the MT that is in contact with the septum.*

If there are suspicions of oesophageal perforation, then an endoscopic should be performed earlier for assessment of the mucosa [17].

To reduce aerodigestive battery ingestion incidences, the Unites States passed the Consumer Product Safety Improvement Act of 2008 to make batteries inaccessible to children 3 years old in toy products. Lately, higher voltage lithium-ion batteries of more than 3 V may mean a potential for greater damage if ingested [18]. Many have advocated for the use of coated batteries, to make them less attractive to children under 3 years of age and to negate any electrical transmission from the battery in the damp and wet environment within the aerodigestive tract [12].

4. Magnetic foreign bodies

Many toys contain whole magnets as a whole (including beads) or fragments of magnets (including ferromagnetic) in varying sizes and shapes. Rare earth magnets such as neodymium have greater strength despite being smaller in size [19]. Magnetic beads are commonly ingested aerodigestive foreign bodies. Magnets taken alone or as 1 unit pose very little risk. However, if several units of magnet are being ingested, this poses a significant danger to the patient. This is because separate units of magnet all pose a north and south pole, and when they come near the other, they may attract one another. The north pole of one magnet may attract the south pole of the other. This may occur when the magnets are next to each other or at different parts of the alimentary tracts with an oesophageal, bowel, or intestinal wall in between.

4.1 Signs and symptoms

Presentations of children with magnetic foreign bodies are non-specific. Several factors play a role such as whether the incident was witnessed or not, the number of magnets ingested, time of incident to presentation, strength of the magnets, and its relative position within the aerodigestive tract.

Magnets attached to each other in a string may impair bowel movement and result in obstruction. Where else, magnet attracted to each other with an intestinal wall or bowel in between may result in localised pressure necrosis, perforation, fistula, sepsis, peritonitis, bowel obstruction, volvulus, and death [20]. In a study done by China over a 3-year period, 14 children presented with magnetic foreign body ingestion. Five children were unwitnessed. Among these five unwitnessed children, all of them presented with intestinal discomfort with intestinal obstruction [21]. The remaining 9 had a history of magnetic ingestion and presented early within 1–8 hours. Only 8 reported intestinal obstructions [21].

4.2 Complications

Complications of multiple magnets ingestion include localised damage, perforation, fistula, and bowel obstruction [12]. Compression of two magnets will inhibit the vascular supply of the surrounding mucosa resulting in ischaemic necrosis. These perforations may be multiple.

4.3 Investigations

Radiographs are reliable in demonstrating metallic objects within the aerodigestive tract. However, the position of the magnet within the abdominal cannot be accurately confirmed from a radiograph. Ultrasound has not been reliable in demonstrating magnetic objects as it is operator-dependent and can be missed [21]. An abdominal radiograph may be misleading at times when two magnets of similar sizes are adhered together, giving the appearance of one. Therefore, two views are often encouraged, and one will need to look hard for a presence of a gap between the radio-opaque foreign body. Abdominal radiographs are also useful to assess for bowel perforation by the presence of pneumoperitoneum or dilated bowels (**Figure 10**) [22]. Both an anterior–posterior view and lateral views of chest and abdominal radiographs have been suggested [19]. If still in doubt, the authors suggest discussing the radiographs with the radiologist. A low-dose limited-field computed tomography (CT) of the abdomen or fluoroscopy can be used as an adjunct if the radiograph and clinical assessment are inconclusive or doubtful respectively. A contrast swallow is not recommended when performing CT scan as it may mask the foreign body [19].

4.4 Management

Treatment will depend on the number of magnets or magnetic units ingested. If only 1 magnet is ingested and the patient being asymptomatic, therefore the wait and watch is acceptable. Time is given for the single magnet to pass through the intestines and defecate. Serial radiographs are encouraged to ascertain the movement of the foreign body with time [22]. If there is one magnet suspected present and shall there be no migration or movement of the foreign body with or without worsening of symptoms, then multiple magnets adhered to each other should be suspected.

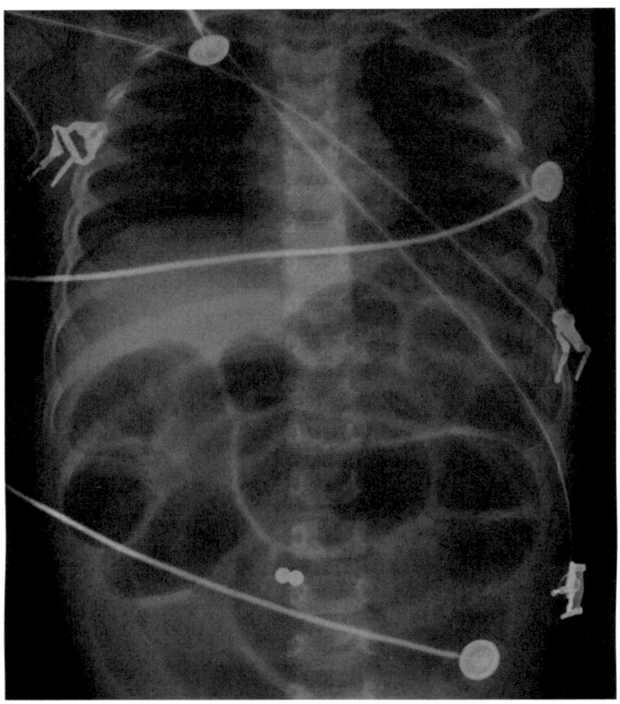

Figure 10.
Diffuse bowel dilatation and two circular radiopaque opacities in the bowel (magnetic beads). No, a small gap between the two beads suggests bowel entrapment between them leading to a perforation.

In the case of multiple magnets, the treatment will depend on the location of the magnets. If the radiograph suggests its position to be within the oesophagus or stomach, an emergency esophagogastroduodenoscopy and removal of the magnets are suggestive. An OGDS will allow for the assessment of the gastric mucosa for necrosis or perforation. If the radiograph is suggestive of a gastric foreign body and the OGDS is negative, perhaps the magnet could have migrated distally. Therefore, duration between radiography and OGDS is time-sensitive. If there are multiple magnets present in the intestines, an emergency laparotomy, either open or laparoscopic, is indicated. Perforations can be inspected, and a bowel resection may need to be performed depending on the assessment.

Some authors have suggested that if multiple magnets form a single stacked object or a string without the entrapment of intestinal mucosa in between and is not scattered, observation with serial radiographs and frequent clinical assessment should be performed. However, this is risky as the string may be altered, forming multiple fragments and be scattered.

5. Conclusion

Non-organic aerodigestive foreign body ingestion is common in children. Button batteries and magnets pose a serious risk of injury and complications. Majority are unwitnessed, requiring a high index of suspicion among children presenting with abdominal discomfort. Urgent removal is indicated.

Author details

Hardip Singh Gendeh[1,2] and Balwant Singh Gendeh[3]*

1 Faculty of Medicine, Department of Otorhinolaryngology, Head and Neck Surgery, Universiti Kebangsaan Malaysia, Kuala Lumpur, Malaysia

2 Allergic Unit, Otorhinolaryngology Clinic, Hospital Canselor Tuanku Muhriz, Kuala Lumpur, Malaysia

3 Pantai Hospital Kuala Lumpur, Kuala Lumpur, Malaysia

*Address all correspondence to: bsgendeh@gmail.com

References

[1] Ekberg O. The cricopharyngeus revisited. The British Journal of Radiology. 1986;**59**(705):875-879. DOI: 10.1259/0007-1285-59-705-875

[2] Passali D, Gregori D, Lorenzoni G, Cocca S, Loglisci M, Passali FM, et al. Foreign body injuries in children: A review. Acta Otorhinolaryngologica Italica. 2015;**35**(4):265-271

[3] Bajaj D, Sachdeva A, Deepak D. Foreign body aspiration. Journal of Thoracic Disease. 2021;**13**(8):5159-5175

[4] Guelfguat M, Kaplinskiy V, Reddy SH, DiPoce J. Clinical guidelines for imaging and reporting ingested foreign bodies. AJR. American Journal of Roentgenology. 2014;**203**(1):37-53

[5] Arabi Mianroodi A, Teimouri Y, Vallance NA. Foreign bodies: Aspirated or ingested? A report of two unusual cases. Iranian Journal of Otorhinolaryngology. 2012;**24**(67):91-94

[6] Gendeh BS, Gendeh HS, Purnima S, Gregori D, Gulati A. Inhaled foreign body impaction: A review of literature in Malaysian children. Indian Journal of Pediatrics. 2019;**86**:2024

[7] Litovitz T, Schmitz BF. Ingestion of cylindrical and button batteries: An analysis of 2382 cases. Pediatrics. 1992;**89**(4):747-757

[8] Sheikh A. Button batteries ingestion in children. Pediatric Emergency Care. 1993;**9**(4):224-229

[9] Thompson N, Lowe-Posford F, Mant TGK, Volans GN. Button battery ingestion: A review. Adverse Drug Reactions and Acute Poisoning Review. 1990;**9**(3):157-180

[10] Lin VY, Daniel SJ, Papsin BC. Button batteries in the ear, nose and upper aerodigestive tract. International Journal of Pediatric Otorhinolaryngology. 2004;**68**(4):473-479

[11] Thabet MH, Basha WM, Askar S. Button battery foreign bodies in children: Hazards, management, and recommendations. BioMed Research International. 2013;**2013**:846091

[12] Laulicht B, Traverso G, Deshpande V, Langer R, Karp JM. Simple battery armor to protect against gastrointestinal injury from accidental ingestion. Proceedings of the National Academy of Sciences of the United States of America. 2014;**111**(46):16490-16495

[13] Litovitz T, Whitaker N, Clark L. Preventing battery ingestions: An analysis of 8648 cases. Pediatrics. 2010;**125**(6):1178-1183

[14] Mubarak A, Benninga MA, Broekaert I, Dolinsek J, Homan M, Mas E, et al. Diagnosis, management, and prevention of button battery ingestion in childhood: A European society for paediatric gastroenterology hepatology and nutrition position paper. Journal of Pediatric Gastroenterology and Nutrition. 2021;**73**(1):129-136

[15] Baharudin N, Gendeh H, Teh HM. Neck radiograph halo sign: Do not be fooled. Cureus. 2023;**15**(4):e38029

[16] Sasitharan P, Mohamad A, Gendeh HS. Button battery ingestion in children—An impending catastrophe. Visual Journal of Emergency Medicine. 2023;**33**(1):1-2

[17] Sethia R, Gibbs H, Jacobs IN, Reilly JS, Rhoades K, Jatana KR.

Current management of button battery injuries. Laryngoscope Investigative Otolaryngology. 2021;**6**(3):549-563

[18] Soccorso G et al. 20 mm lithium button battery causing an oesophageal perforation in a toddler: Lessons in diagnosis and treatment. Archives of Disease in Childhood. 2012;**97**(8):746-747

[19] Otjen JP, Rohrmann CA Jr, Iyer RS. Imaging pediatric magnet ingestion with surgical-pathological correlation. Pediatric Radiology. 2013;**43**(7):851-859

[20] Lin A, Chan LCN, Hon KLE, Tsui SYB, Pang KKY, Cheung HM, et al. Magnetic foreign body ingestion in children: The attractive hazards. Case Reports in Pediatrics. 2019;**2019**:3549242

[21] Huang YK, Hong SX, Tai IH, et al. Clinical characteristics of magnetic foreign body misingestion in children. Scientific Reports. 2021;**11**:18680

[22] Kircher MF, Milla S, Callahan MJ. Ingestion of magnetic foreign bodies causing multiple bowel perforations. Pediatric Radiology. 2007;**37**(9):933-936

Section 2

Airway Foreign Body

Chapter 4

Foreign Body in the Airway

Varun tej Gonuguntla, Amnah Khalid and Muhammad Perwaiz

Abstract

Foreign Body (FB) aspiration incidence follows a bimodal distribution and is commonly seen in children under the age of 5 or adults with advanced age. The type of FB can be organic or non-organic and varies depending on age, region of the world, and socioeconomic status. In children, FB aspiration is often a consequence of development and exploration. Aspiration of FB in adults typically occurs when cough reflex is blunted due to altered sensorium (from drugs, medications, advanced age), trauma to the airway, poor swallowing, or anatomical variations in the GI tract (strictures, Zenker's Diverticulum, etc. Symptoms can range from cough to asphyxiation depending on the acuity of the aspiration event. Initial management is focused on ensuring there is no airway compromise leading to respiratory failure. Bronchoscopy is the treatment of choice to retrieve the FB. This chapter will review the incidence of FB aspiration in children vs. adults and will focus on diagnosis and treatment including bronchoscopy, role of ECMO, and surgical intervention.

Keywords: foreign body, aspiration, cough, chest radiograph, bronchoscopy, anesthesia

1. Introduction

Foreign Body (FB) aspiration incidence is commonly seen in children or adults with advanced age [1, 2]. It is one of the most common reasons for emergency department visits and as of 2017, FB aspiration with asphyxiation is one of the leading causes of death in infants and fourth most common cause of death among preschool children [3]. The incidence of FB aspiration in children is higher than adults and it is more common in males than females [4–9]. According to some studies, up to 80% of FB aspiration cases are seen in kids less than three years of age with peak incidence below 1–2 years of age [10–14].

The type of FB can be organic or non-organic and varies depending on age, region of the world, and socioeconomic status. In children, FB aspiration is often a consequence of development and exploration. Young children tend to explore objects by placing them in their mouths and accidental aspiration results in FB in the airway. Furthermore, swallowing involves delicate coordination of oropharynx and the gastrointestinal tract. In children, the swallowing mechanism is not well developed and asynchrony between actions such as crying, laughing, or breathing while eating results in aspiration into the airway more easily.

Adults have a developed cough and swallow reflex which induces a strong cough to expel the FB out of the airway. Aspiration of FB in adult typically occurs when this reflex is blunted due to altered sensorium (from drugs, medications, advanced age), trauma to the airway, poor swallowing, or anatomical variations in the GI tract (strictures, Zenker's Diverticulum, etc). In adults, organic objects such as food is the most common FB that is aspirated. The type of food that is aspirated has a geographical variation and the type of cuisine that is available. In the western countries it is usually nuts such as peanuts, whereas in the southeast Asian countries it is typically bone fragments (from chicken, fish, etc) [15–17]. There are also cases of iatrogenic foreign bodies especially in the healthcare setting such as medical equipment that is accidentally dislodged into the airway. For example, there are reports of oral care equipment dislodged into the airway, pieces of bronchoscope, biopsy forceps, cytology brushes, and blood clots from airway blee ding [2, 17, 18].

2. Clinical presentation

Cough is the most common symptom with up to 96% of the patients reporting this after FB aspiration. The symptoms depend on the acuity of the aspiration, the type of FB that is aspirated, and location of FB in the airway. Acute aspiration of FB in the upper airway can either cause complete obstruction or partial obstruction. Common symptoms of partial obstruction are cough, wheezing, chest pain, and dyspnea [19]. Complete obstruction typically presents as stridor, hoarseness, choking and cyanosis. If the FB is in the smaller airways, the typical symptoms are cough and wheezing.

However, in up to 36% of the cases, the patients can have silent aspiration and can be asymptomatic. These patients could present with chronic symptoms such as cough, recurrent infections and further work up might show aspirated foreign bodies. Despite the high prevalence, FB aspirations are difficult to diagnose. A detailed history is key to diagnosis, especially a history of a choking event should increase suspicion for foreign body aspiration (FBA). Clinical presentation can vary from subtle respiratory symptoms to life threatening airway compromise. In children, if the aspiration event is not witnessed by a caregiver, the diagnosis can be delayed. In up to 50% of cases, initial symptoms of choking, cough, dyspnea can resolve within minutes and result in a symptom-free interval. These children present later with non-specific symptoms including chronic cough and recurrent pneumonias [20]. A child presenting with cyanosis, altered mental status and or severe respiratory distress is indicative of complete or near complete airway obstruction and requires immediate intervention [21].

The most common presenting symptom in children is acute onset of cough but other signs and symptoms include tachypnea, dyspnea, stridor, wheeze, hemoptysis, hoarse voice, fever, chest, and throat pain [21]. Physical findings include wheeze, cough, stridor, rales, and decreased breath sounds [21]. Stridor is heard with inspiration and can indicate obstruction above the level of the thoracic inlet. Expiratory wheeze is heard with obstruction below the level of the thoracic inlet, and unilateral wheeze can indicate the general site of obstruction [21].

3. Diagnostic workup

Chest radiographs are performed as part of the initial workup. They are not recommended to rule out FBA. Chest radiographs may not show the aspirated FB in 25% of cases. Chest radiographs can have secondary signs that may assist with diagnosis. These include air trapping or obstructive emphysema due to ball-valve effect of the FB in the bronchus. Chest radiographs may also show atelectasis, pneumonia, pneumothorax and pneumomediastinum. Films obtained in forced expiration and inspiration can highlight these signs. These may be difficult to obtain in younger children and thus lateral films can help reveal such signs when the impacted lung is in the dependent position [21]. Computed tomography of the chest is another option. Though more specific, its use is limited to the cooperation of the patient, use of sedation and increased radiation [21]. Definite diagnosis and treatment is bronchoscopy accompanied by removal of the FB with the appropriate instruments. Blood in the airway, increased airway secretions, granulation tissue or pneumonia may impair bronchoscopy visualization of the FB.

4. Airway

The approach to management of pediatric FB aspiration will depend on whether the obstruction is partial or complete and the level of consciousness [22].

Children who can cough, cry or speak have an incomplete airway obstruction. These patients are managed expectantly, as attempts to relieve the partial obstruction may dislodge the FB and worsen the degree of obstruction. When the patient shows signs of tiring or is progressing toward complete obstruction, removal should be considered. Attempts to remove the FB should be made in the operating room. Sedation with ketamine (1-2 mg/kg IV or 4 mg/kg IM) produces dissociation while maintain respiratory drive and airway reflexes. Once sedated, laryngoscope is inserted with anatomic visualization to identify any supraglottic FB [22].

A complete airway obstruction is indicated by loss of ability to phonate or cough. Chest wall movement persists with attempted respiratory efforts. Pediatric basic life support techniques should be used in the conscious patient with complete airway obstruction. The increased intrathoracic pressure is expected to expel the FB from the airway. In infants, this is done with child in a head down position, using cycles of back blows and chest compressions. In children older than 1 year, the Heimlich maneuver is recommended. The oropharynx should be examined first for a visible FB. If no FB is visualized, laryngoscopy can be attempted in the emergency department. A neuromuscular blocking agent is only recommended if the child has a clenched mouth other signs of muscle tone that is prohibiting the laryngoscopy. If a FB is identified, removal is attempted using Magill or alligator forceps. This should be done with caution as to avoid advancing the FB to a position where it becomes more tightly dislodged or unretrievable. If BLS and laryngoscopy are unsuccessful, the FB should be advanced distally into either mainstem bronchus using a stylet or endotracheal tube. The "lip to tip" distance should be measured using the Broselow-Luten tape or other formulas. The child would be intubated with the endotracheal tube and stylet advanced as deeply as possible. This should result in advanced of the obstructing material into the mainstem bronchus usually the right. The endotracheal tube should then be withdrawn back to the previously measured distance. This maneuver should allow ventilation through one lung. If increased resistance develops subsequently, organic material may have dislodged and obstructed the endotracheal tube tip. Replacement of the endotracheal tube using the appropriate insertion depth is performed [22].

Short acting agents are preferred for induction and maintenance of anesthesia as depth of anesthesia can be rapidly adapted to the procedure requirements. A percutaneous approach is rarely indicated in FB aspiration. Needle cricothyrotomy will only be successful if the needle entry site is distal to the obstruction. If the FB is not visualized during laryngoscopy attempts, it is unlikely that the percutaneous approach will be distal to the object. Once the airway is secured after forced intubation or needle cricothyrotomy, the patient should be taken to the operating room for removal of the FB with a bronchoscope or thoracotomy [22].

In adults, similar challenges are encountered with partially or completely obstructed airway. In partially obstructed airway, any action or failure to take specific action can results into converting the partially obstructed airway into a completely obstructed. When a complete obstruction is present, bag-mask ventilation or insertion of extra glottic device can worsen the situation by dislodging the obstruction from supraglottic to below the vocal cords. Endotracheal intubation with bag ventilation may also result in a complete inability to move any air. Signs of incomplete airway obstruction in an adult patient include stridor, altered phonation, subjective difficulty breathing and sense of fear or panic [22].

Management of airway obstruction depends on the location of the FB and whether the obstruction is incomplete or complete. The location may be supraglottic, infraglottic or distal to the carina. In an incomplete FB obstruction where the patient is breathing spontaneously and saturating adequately, efforts should be made to plan for prompt removal in the operating room (OR). Emergency airway equipment should be immediately accessible in case the patient deteriorates. If transfer to an OR is not possible then decision for removal in the emergency department must be made. The first step may involve handing the patient a rigid suction device to attempt self-retrieval. If this fails, the next step is to attempt laryngoscopy. The patient should be preoxygenated and given topical anesthesia. A dissociative agent or titrate sedation should only be used if needed. The patient is placed semi supine, anesthetized and the laryngoscope is inserted with careful inspection at each level so as not to dislodge the FB. if the patient is unable to tolerate a semi supine position, laryngoscopy can be attempted with the patient sitting up. A flexible endoscope, inserted through the nose, can also be used to visualize the FB. Once identified, the instrument for removal is selected based on the characteristics of the FB. Once successfully removed, a repeat laryngoscopy should be performed to ensure no remaining particulate. The patient should be observed until recovered from anesthesia and based on clinical symptoms [22].

In complete airway obstruction the patient is unable to breathe or phonate and appears terrified. Oxygen saturation usually falls rapidly resulting in loss of consciousness. Initial management is determined by level of consciousness. If the patient is conscious, back slaps and then abdominal thrusts (such as Heimlich Maneuver) are recommended in the latest guidelines by the Internal Liason Committee on Resuscitation. If available, non-invasive anti-choking devices (such as LiveVac) can also be used. However, these devices should not be used first line as they can result in delay in treatment. If the abdominal thrust are unsuccessful, cardiopulmonary resuscitation chest thrusts should be initiated especially if loss of consciousness or impending cardiorespiratory arrest. At this point, immediate direct or video laryngoscopy should be performed. Bag mask ventilation should not be attempted before laryngoscopy for risk of dislodgement of the FB from supraglottic to infraglottic position [22].

Supraglottic obstructing FB is easily identified by direct/video laryngoscopy. A suitable instrument can be used to remove the FB. The patient may begin to ventilate spontaneously. If this does not occur, immediate intubation and positive pressure ventilation is initiated. If the FB is visualized but cannot be removed cricothyroidotomy should be performed to establish an airway. If no FB is identified by laryngoscopy, the patient should be intubated and ventilated. Resistance with bag ventilation through the endotracheal tube indicates complete obstruction of the trachea [22].

Complete FB airway obstruction in the trachea requires three techniques. The first is to remove the FB with vigorous suction. After intubation, a neonatal meconium aspirator may be directly attached to the ETT and then connected to wall suction. For foreign bodies larger than the endotracheal lumen, both the tube and the FB are removed together with continuous suction. The patient is then reintubated. If this fails, the third technique is applied. This involves pushing the FB into a mainstem bronchus by advancing the ETT and then withdrawing it into the mid-trachea, thus allowing ventilation of one lung. If all above mentioned techniques are not successful, the patient either has a one mainstem bronchus obstruction and a tension pneumothorax on the other side. As a result, bilateral needle thoracostomy is performed as it is unclear which airway was obstructed. In the case that there is no pneumothorax, the only clinical possibility is that there is a bilateral mainstem obstruction from which survival is not possible [22].

5. Bronchoscopy

5.1 Rigid bronchoscopy

Bronchoscopy has become the standard of diagnosis and treatment for FB aspiration. The use of flexible versus rigid bronchoscopy depends on patient age, local resources, and expertise. Rigid bronchoscopy is usually required for successful removal of foreign bodies in children. FB aspiration (FBA) is most seen in the young and elderly. There are many risk factors that have been associated with this including alcohol intoxication, sedative/hypnotic drug use, poor dentition, senility, primary neurologic disorders with impairment of swallowing or mental status, seizures, Parkinson's disease, general anesthesia and Zenker's diverticulum. A detailed history and physical examination along with chest imaging are necessary [23].

Rigid bronchoscopy is the therapeutic instrument of choice for the airway. Its large size and stiff construction allow the endoscopist to access and manipulate the trachea and right and left proximal airways. Indications for rigid bronchoscopy include large tissue biopsies, removal of complex foreign bodies, management of massive hemoptysis and therapeutic interventions for intrinsic and extrinsic airway obstruction [23].

There are three components of a rigid bronchoscope: barrel, multifunction head and telescope/light source. There are two main types of scopes: rigid bronchoscopes and rigid tracheoscopes. Rigid bronchoscopes are longer and have side ventilation fenestrations allowing them to access the right and left bronchial tree. The barrel is a hollow metal tube with a beveled distal tip which helps with lifting the tongue and epiglottis and allows passage between vocal cords. The proximal end of the scope attaches to the multifunction head permitting ventilation and instrument access. The light source attaches to the proximal end of the scope or to the telescope lens. The inner diameter of the adult rigid bronchoscope ranges form 7-13 mm and outer diameter from 8 to 14 mm. larger scopes can accommodate larger stents and address tracheal and mainstem pathology. Smaller scopes are more suitable for distal left and right mainstem bronchi and up till bronchus intermedius pathology. Ancillary equipment including rigid forceps, suction catheters, stent, and stent deployers, scalpel, scissors, balloons, mechanical dilators, endoscopic resectors should be present [23].

Intubating a patient with the rigid bronchoscopy require appropriate sedation and proper patient positioning. Sedation and the use of paralytics depend on the clinical stability of the patient. The rigid construction of the scope requires straight and direct access to the larynx. The patient is positioned supine with either a towel roll under the shoulders or the head of bed should be dropped allowing the neck to maximally extended. This allows a more linear route through the vocal cords by elevating the larynx. The oral, pharyngeal and laryngeal axis should be aligned anteriorly in order to access the trachea. The bronchoscope is then used to intubate the trachea and advanced under direct visualization either directly down the barrel or through the telescope and camera optics [23].

The most common anatomic site for aspirated foreign bodies is the right bronchial tree due to the shorter and wider right main bronchus and anatomic angle. Initial attempt at FB extraction with flexible bronchoscopy is reasonable but prompt conversion to rigid bronchoscopy can prevent complications and need for surgical intervention. In cases of unstable airway due to FB aspiration, rigid bronchoscopy is the first tool of choice for extraction and management. In a retrospective study in 60 adults presents with FB aspiration, rigid bronchoscopy had a success rate of 96% while flexible bronchoscopy was successful in 61% of cases. In children, it is the preferred treatment method for FB extraction. In a prospective study evaluating the role of rigid and flexible bronchoscopes in children, determined that clinical and radiologic findings were useful in deciding between the two methods. The study reported that rigid bronchoscopes must be used if there is asphyxia, a radio-opaque FB in radiography and decreased air sounds along with obstructive overinflation in the chest radiograph [24].

The larger diameter of the rigid bronchoscope allows bronchoscopist to manage foreign bodies of varying size, shape and texture. The luminal diameter of the scope dictates only the size of the working instrument which will grasp and manipulate the FB. The FB, grasper and scope can be removed en masse if necessary to recover the FB.

In 2022 Han et al., reported 99.2% success rate of FB removal with flexible bronchoscopy. They reported the use of rigid bronchoscopy in only five of the cases [25]. In a meta-analysis published by Chantzaras et al. of 23 papers published between 2001 an d2021, in 2588 cases flexible bronchoscopy was successful in 87.1% of cases [26].

5.2 Flexible bronchoscopy

Bronchoscopy is the gold standard diagnostic and therapeutic intervention in management of FB aspiration in the airway. Rigid bronchoscope was first used by Dr. Gustave Killian in 1897 to remove a FB (bone) from main bronchus. It has remained the mainstay bronchoscopy technique especially in management of FB for almost 70 years until invention of fiberoptic bronchoscope by Shigeto Ikeda in 1968. Since its invention, it has expanded the therapeutic options available for management of FB removal [27–31].

Flexible bronchoscopy is able to navigate to distal airways due to its flexibility as well as length increasing the ability for smaller and more distal foreign bodies to be visualized and extracted. Therefore, it should be considered in every patient with concern for FB aspiration into airway to perform thorough examination of the entire airway. In many instances, the FB might not be seen on the chest imaging and bronchoscopy allows for direct visualization of the object and to see if it is causing obstruction of airways. Especially in chronic aspiration, there could be inflammatory changes and granulomatous reaction making the foreign object difficult to discern in imaging.

There are several accessories available for therapeutic management of FB aspiration in the airway that can be used with flexible bronchoscopy. The choice depends on various factors such as type of FB, consistency, location in the airway, and shape. Some of the accessories are similar to those used in other subspecialities such as Gastroenterology, Urology, and Interventional radiology. These tools will be discussed in detail below:

5.2.1 Forceps

Forceps that are used in flexible bronchoscopes come in different cup sizes, shapes, rotation mechanism, central fenestration or needles, or presence or absence of "teeth". The forceps can be used for biopsy or for grasping objects such as foreign bodies. The biopsy forceps have a central scooping in the cup with or without central spike and with or without teeth to allow for tissue removal (**Figure 1**). Grasping forceps allow you to grip onto an object to remove it. Grasping forceps include three-pronged, alligator jaw, rat-tooth, shark-tooth, W-shaped, and rubber tip grasping forceps (**Figure 2**).

The specific use of these grasping forceps depends on the type of FB. For example, in hard FBs rat-tooth, alligator-jaw, or shark-tooth are the most common forceps used as they provide a good grasp of the object due to their teeth. If the FB has smooth edges, or sharp edges, rubber tip forceps can help obtain better grasp on the object while minimizing damage to the surrounding structures (**Figure 2**). W-shaped and V-shaped damage to the surrounding structures (**Figure 1**). W-shaped and V-shaped forceps allow for more delicate maneuvers and allow to grasp a large FB because of

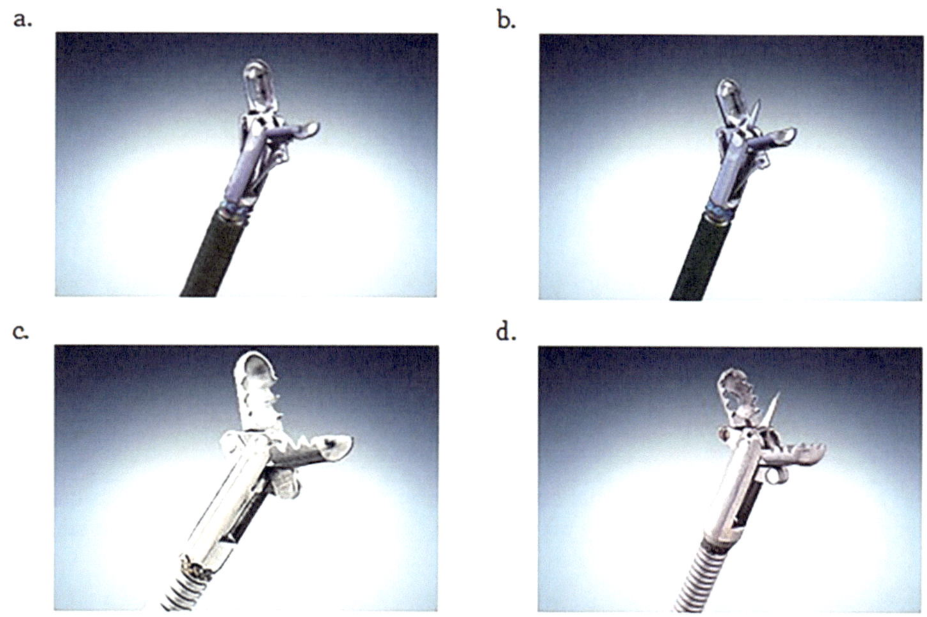

Figure 1.
Biopsy Forceps in Bronchoscopy. a. Biopsy forceps with curved cup with ability to grasp and remove tissue; b. Biopsy forceps with central needle which enhances tissue collection; c. Biopsy Forceps with alligator jaw (jagged edges) allows tearing of tissue d. Biopsy Forceps with alligator jaw and central needle.

a. b. c. d. e. f.

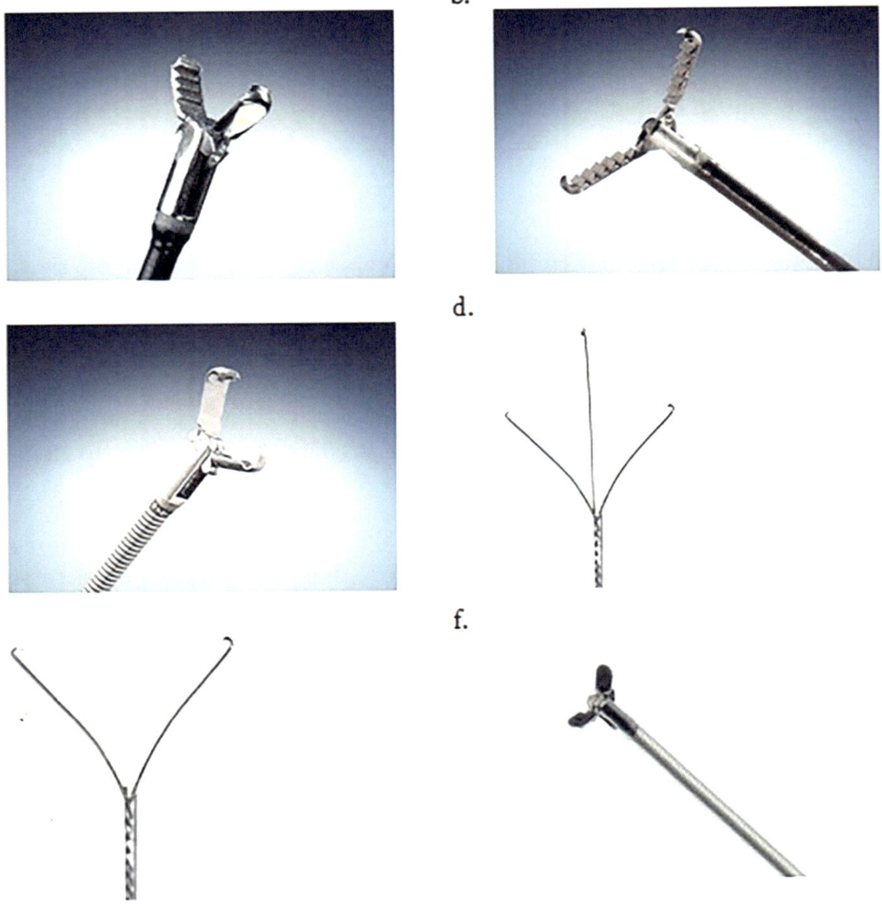

Figure 2.
Grasping Forceps in Bronchoscopy. a. Alligator Jaw; b. Rat-Tooth Jaw; c. Shark Tooth Jaw; d. Three-pronged; e. W-shaped; f. Rubber Tipped.

their large cup opening width. Typically, grasping forceps are best suitable for inorganic/organic foreign objects with hard consistency (coins, nails, bones, etc). Other tools might be better suited for organic objects which will be discussed below.

5.2.2 Baskets

They are used for objects that are large, have irregular contours, or friable objects that are difficult to grasp. There are different types of baskets: some with a central net and some without which will be explained in detail below (**Figure 3**).

5.2.2.1 Dormia basket

It was invented by Italian Urologist, Dormia and has since been used by Gastroenterologists and Urologists to retrieve stones in the common bile duct or ureters. The basket is encapsulated by a Teflon catheter and when it is advanced into the

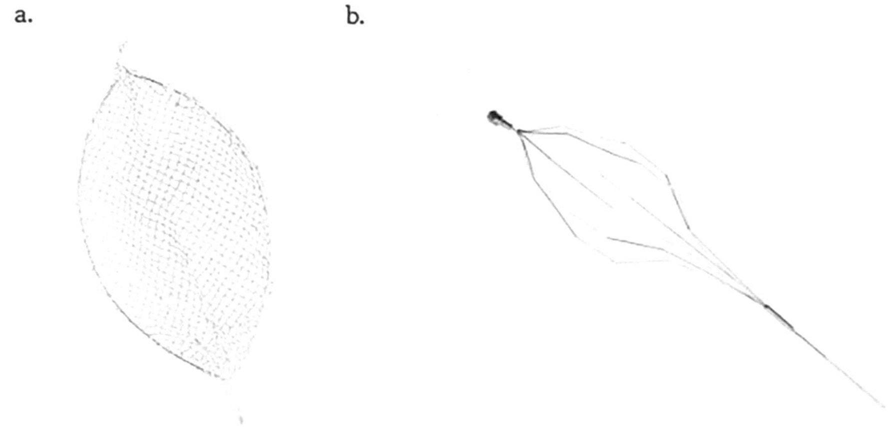

Figure 3.
Grasping Baskets vs Fishnet Baskets. a. Alligator Jaw; b. Rat-Tooth Jaw; c. Shark Tooth Jaw; d. Three-pronged; e. W-shaped; f. Rubber Tipped.

airway, its wings (flexible loops of metal) open exposing the basket which is maneuvered to capture the FB. The basket is then retrieved back to the catheter to close the basket around the FB. The FB is usually larger than the channel of bronchoscopy.

5.2.2.2 Fishnet basket

It is a modified version of a polypectomy snare, in which a mesh of thin thread is attached to the snare wire for easy folding and unfolding. It is helpful in retrieving large friable FB such as organic food material [31].

5.2.2.3 Grasping baskets

They have multiple wings that flare when advanced out of the sheath with space between them that can be used to trap rounded edges that are difficult to grasp with forceps [32, 33].

5.2.2.4 Snares

These are flexible wings without central mesh in between that can also be used. However, they are very difficult to maneuver in the airway and grasp onto an object so they are rarely used in FB removal [34].

5.2.3 Balloon catheters

Inflatable balloon catheters are one of the most underutilized tools in FB removal. These catheters are long tubular structures with distal balloon that can be inflated such as Fogarty catheter. This allows for the catheter to bypass the obstruction. The balloon is inflated distal to the obstruction and the FB can be pulled out of the airway slowly along with the FB slowly. This tool can be helpful in dislodging partially occluded FB more proximally and can even help in complete obstruction of airway from FB that is difficult to grasp.

5.2.4 Cryoprobe

The cryoprobe was first developed to freeze endotracheal or endobronchial tumor by Gage in 1968. Its use has since been expanded to include transbronchial tissue biopsy and FB removal. There is more literature in its use as an alternative to surgical lung biopsy in interstitial lung disease (ILD) and has even been included as part of guidelines in management of ILD if they are performed by an expert proceduralist.

Similarly, it is also used in the removal of FB. The cryotherapy system consists of cryogen, cryoconsole, and cryoprobe. Typical cryogens are nitric oxide or nitrogen which then undergo rapid gas- decompression in the cryoconsole which generates extremely low temperatures of -15C to -40C in the cryoprobe tip which is used to freeze and adhere to objects with water content such as human tissue and can then be pulled along with the probe. Therefore, it is extremely efficient in removing foreign objects that are rich in water content (food, blood clots, mucous balls, etc). The object can adhere to the cryoprobe tip and can be removed [35]. However, extreme caution should be maintained in making sure that the cryoprobe is not close to the mucosa when removing FB so that it does not inadvertently injure the mucosa.

5.2.5 Magnet extractor

It has a flexible probe with a magnetic cylinder at its tip and can be used for metallic foreign objects. It is especially useful in iatrogenic FBs such as broken cytology brushes, forceps biopsy tips, guidewires, etc. [36, 37].

5.2.6 Laser beam

Objects that cannot be removed by any of the techniques listed above or rigid bronchoscopy, LASER beam can be used to break it down into smaller pieces which can then be extracted. The neodymium-yttrium-aluminum-garnet (Nd:YAG) laser is the most commonly used type of laser. There are cases of LASER beam being used in breakdown of an aspirated chicken bone which was then retrieved using biopsy forceps [38]. Similarly, there are other reports of two patients where LASER beam is used in removal of thumbtacks [39]. It can cause airway fire similar to cautery tools and argon plasma tools in the airway, so anesthesia should be made aware that when using the laser beam, to decrease exhaled FiO_2 to <30%.

5.2.7 Complications

5.2.7.1 Bleeding

Bleeding is an expected complication from removal of FB. Organic FBs are known to cause mucosal irritation and the degree of damage depends on the type of the agent swallowed. For example, inorganic objects such as iron pills are extremely caustic with quick mucosal irritation and with prolonged exposure to mucosa can form ulceration and strictures which can bleed when attempting to remove. In some institutions, it is common practice to use a short course of steroids before removal of FB especially if it is a chronic FB to help with the inflammation [40, 41].

Therefore, it is important to make sure that one is prepared with tools to deal with massive hemorrhage. The proceduralist must have a rigid bronchoscope available as it is easier to manage hemoptysis using rigid bronchoscope. Other tools such as cold saline, epinephrine, thrombin, electrocautery, and APC must be readily available for usage in these critical situations.

5.2.7.2 Dislodging FB

It is possible that when performing examination with bronchoscopy, manipulation of the airway can dislodge the FB which can cause the object to fall deeper into the airway causing further obstruction. If this dislodgement happens in proximal trachea it can lead to asphyxiation and can lead to cardiac arrest. Therefore, the inspection of the airway must be done carefully. In some institutions, in cases of partial obstruction from FB, the proceduralist may insert catheter and balloon distal to the FB and use the balloon to prevent dislodgement and use it to pull the object more proximal into the trachea.

Furthermore, in cases where the FB is large, it is important to have a tight grip on the accessory used to retrieve the FB and pull the accessory into the bronchoscope as much as possible and remove the accessory and bronchoscope together with complete visualization of the FB. This must be done with FBs that are sharp to make sure no mucosal or airway injury.

5.2.7.3 Other complications

Mortality rates of bronchoscopy for foreign bodies in children vary from 0.1% to 3.4%. Complications associated with bronchoscopy in children include failure to remove the FB, hypoxemia, laryngeal edema, and pneumothorax [42]. In a retrospective analysis done by Powers et al. on 2302 cases of FBA in children who underwent bronchoscopy, the most common comorbidity was structural pulmonary abnormality (10.5%) followed by sepsis (6.7%) and Asthma (6.5%). The overall rate of complication post bronchoscopy was low. Pneumonia (0.8%) was the highest followed by reintubation (0.4%). Intraoperative bleeding was seen in 4 patients (0.2%) and one patient (0.04%) experienced cardiac arrest and required CPR. Overall mortality rate was 0.4% within 30 days after bronchoscopy [43].

5.3 Flexible bronchoscopy vs rigid bronchoscopy

Flexible bronchoscopy can be just as successful in retrieval of FB as rigid bronchoscopy. According to a retrospective study by Sehgal et al., the success rate of flexible bronchoscopy in the removal of FB is as high as 92% [29]. The success rate is higher up to 97–99% when both rigid and flexible bronchoscopy are used in tandem [40]. Rigid bronchoscopy success rate ranges from 86 to 100%. Rigid bronchoscopy is better suited for FBs that are in larger proximal airways such as trachea or mainstem bronchi as they are easier to visualize and navigate to. FBs that are in distal airways typically need flexible bronchoscopy. However, the data varies between studies and this variability can be due to the experience of the proceduralist and the experience of the institution where the procedure is being performed. There are numerous reports of FB removal failure from rigid bronchoscopy but was successful via flexible bronchoscopy and vice versa.

In a study by Ng et al., they looked at the rate of successful FB removal between flexible bronchoscopy and rigid bronchoscopy. Flexible bronchoscopy was successful in 80% of the cases compared to 100% success rate in rigid bronchoscopy [44]. Further study of patients where flexible bronchoscopy failed showed that rigid bronchoscopy was better in patients with no comorbidities, delay in FB aspiration diagnosis, and hard FBs. The correct modality of bronchoscopy depends on FB, the location in the airway and ultimately the experience and comfort of the proceduralist.

6. ECMO

There has been growing body of literature where extracorporeal membrane oxygenation (ECMO) has been used in cases of refractory respiratory failure in the setting of FB aspiration [45–50]. It originated from the invention and use of cardiopulmonary bypass in the OR. The Cardiopulmonary bypass was first successfully used in human in 1953 and initially involved use of "bubble" oxygenators where oxygen is bubbled through a reservoir of blood to create blood-gas interface and gas exchange [51]. It was later replaced by membrane oxygenators where there is separation of respiratory gases from blood making long term use of these devices possible. In 1972, Dr. Hill and colleagues used a membrane oxygenator to administer ECMO for extended periods outside the operating room. Further progress since then allowed its use in situations involving respiratory failure [52].

There are two types of ECMO, there is VV-ECMO (veno-venous ECMO) which provides respiratory support and VA-ECMO (veno-arterial ECMO) which provides cardiac and respiratory support. ECMO circuit is rather simple in its components and consists of mechanical pump, oxygenator, and a heat exchanger which is inserted into the patient [53].

In cases of FB aspiration, there are complications that arise such as complete occlusion of airway with inability to ventilate patient, pulmonary edema, bleeding, acute respiratory distress syndrome, and severe lung injury which can result in severe hypoxemic respiratory failure [48, 54]. ECMO was also used in cases where the FB is small particles such as sand or saw dust making the extraction difficult. In other cases, there may be resource limitation with limited access to rigid bronchoscopy or situations where bronchoscopic interventions fail and VV-ECMO can be used as a "bridging" therapy until further curative treatment can be performed.

According to a study by Anton-Martin et al., who studied ECMO use in children across 251 institutions with FB aspiration, it has been used in more than 10 cases. In all these cases, ECMO allowed for prolonged respiratory support and in this cohort, they reported survival of >90% [55]. Similarly, another study by Park et al., where they studied ECMO use in children where respiratory instability led to inability to perform bronchoscopy. ECMO allowed for stabilization with eventual bronchoscopic intervention with complete recovery of patients [56]. These case studies show that in institutions where there is no provider with expertise to perform bronchoscopic intervention, patients are too unstable, or institutions where there is easy ECMO access, it could be used as a rescue therapy for patients with FB aspiration with critical airway compromise to avoid respiratory arrest.

7. Surgical management

As mentioned prior, Bronchoscopy is the gold standard and the most successful option for removal of FB in the airway with success rates as high as 98%. However, in situations where endoscopic and bronchoscopic interventions fail or patients have trauma to the viscera due to penetrating trauma from the FB, or long-term complication with failure to remove the FB, then surgery could be considered. Surgical options such as tracheostomy, thoracotomy, bronchotomy, or lung resection might be needed to remove FB [57–60].

Abbreviations

FB	foreign body
OR	operating room
ETT	endotracheal tube

Author details

Varun tej Gonuguntla, Amnah Khalid and Muhammad Perwaiz*
Icahn School of Medicine at Mount Sinai, United States of America

*Address all correspondence to: perwaizm1@nychhc.org

References

[1] Rose D, Dubensky L. Airway foreign bodies. [updated 2023 Aug 7]. In: StatPearls [Internet]. Treasure Island (FL): StatPearls Publishing; 2023. Available from: https://www.ncbi.nlm.nih.gov/books/NBK539756/

[2] Blanco Ramos M, Botana-Rial M, García-Fontán E, Fernández-Villar A, Gallas TM. Update in the extraction of airway foreign bodies in adults. Journal of Thoracic Disease. 2016;**8**(11):3452-3456. DOI: 10.21037/jtd.2016.11.32

[3] Salih AM, Alfaki M, Alam-Elhuda DM. Airway foreign bodies: A critical review for a common pediatric emergency. World Journal of Emergency Medicine. 2016;**7**(1):5-12. DOI: 10.5847/wjem.j.1920-8642.2016.01.001

[4] Rodríguez H, Cuestas G, Botto H, et al. Complications in children from foreign bodies in the airway. Acta Otorrinolaringológica Española. 2016;**67**(2):93-101. DOI: 10.1016/j.otorri.2015.01.003

[5] Shivakumar AM, Naik AS, Prashanth KB, Shetty KD, Praveen DS. Tracheobronchial foreign bodies. Indian Journal of Pediatrics. 2003;**70**(10):793-797. DOI: 10.1007/BF02723797

[6] Cohen SR, Herbert WI, Lewis GB Jr, Geller KA. Foreign bodies in the airway. Five-year retrospective study with special reference to management. The Annals of Otology, Rhinology, and Laryngology. 1980;**89**(5 Pt 1):437-442. DOI: 10.1177/000348948008900513

[7] Kaur K, Sonkhya N, Bapna AS. Foreign bodies in the tracheobronchial tree: A prospective study of fifty cases. Indian Journal of Otolaryngology and Head & Neck Surgery. 2002;**54**(1):30-34. DOI: 10.1007/BF02911002

[8] Hughes CA, Baroody FM, Marsh BR. Pediatric tracheobronchial foreign bodies: Historical review from the Johns Hopkins Hospital. The Annals of Otology, Rhinology, and Laryngology. 1996;**105**(7):555-561. DOI: 10.1177/000348949610500712

[9] Shlizerman L, Mazzawi S, Rakover Y, Ashkenazi D. Foreign body aspiration in children: The effects of delayed diagnosis. American Journal of Otolaryngology. 2010;**31**(5):320-324. DOI: 10.1016/j.amjoto.2009.03.007

[10] Ciftci AO, Bingöl-Koloğlu M, Senocak ME, Tanyel FC, Büyükpamukçu N. Bronchoscopy for evaluation of foreign body aspiration in children. Journal of Pediatric Surgery. 2003;**38**(8):1170-1176. DOI: 10.1016/s0022-3468(03)00263-x

[11] Reilly JS, Cook SP, Stool D, Rider G. Prevention and management of aerodigestive foreign body injuries in childhood. Pediatric Clinics of North America. 1996;**43**(6):1403-1411. DOI: 10.1016/s0031-3955(05)70525-3

[12] Committee on Injury, Violence, and Poison Prevention; Prevention of Choking Among Children. Pediatrics. March 2010;**125**(3):601-607. DOI: 10.1542/peds.2009-2862

[13] Yadav SP, Singh J, Aggarwal N, Goel A. Airway foreign bodies in children: Experience of 132 cases. Singapore Medical Journal. 2007;**48**(9):850-853

[14] Brkić F, Umihanić S. Tracheobronchial foreign bodies in children. Experience at ORL clinic Tuzla, 1954-2004. International Journal of Pediatric Otorhinolaryngology.

2007;**71**(6):909-915. DOI: 10.1016/j.ijporl.2007.02.019

[15] Baharloo F, Veyckemans F, Francis C, Biettlot MP, Rodenstein DO. Tracheobronchial foreign bodies: Presentation and management in children and adults. Chest. 1999;**115**(5):1357-1362. DOI: 10.1378/chest.115.5.1357

[16] Patel S, Kazerooni EA. Case 31: foreign body aspiration--chicken vertebra. Radiology 2001;**218**(2):523-525. DOI: 10.1148/radiology.218.2.r01fe49523

[17] Tenda ED, Yakub A, Pitoyo CW, Fardizza F. Combination of bronchoscopic cryoextraction and argon plasma coagulation in treatment of total central airway obstruction caused by giant blood clot formation in massive airway bleeding. Respiratory Medicine Case Reports. 2016;**19**:9-11. Published 2016 Jun 13. DOI: 10.1016/j.rmcr.2016.06.002

[18] Paradis TJ, Dixon J, Tieu BH. The role of bronchoscopy in the diagnosis of airway disease. Journal of Thoracic Disease. 2016;**8**(12):3826-3837. DOI: 10.21037/jtd.2016.12.68

[19] Lan RS. Non-asphyxiating tracheobronchial foreign bodies in adults. The European Respiratory Journal. 1994;**7**(3):510-514. DOI: 10.1183/09031936.94.07030510

[20] Ezer SS, Oguzkurt P, Ince E, Temiz A, Çalıskan E, Hicsonmez A. Foreign body aspiration in children: Analysis of diagnostic criteria and accurate time for bronchoscopy. Pediatric Emergency Care. 2011;**27**(8):723-726. DOI: 10.1097/PEC.0b013e318226c896

[21] Goldfarb S, Piccione J. Diagnostic and Interventional Bronchoscopy in Children. 1st edition 2021. Switzerland: Springer International Publishing AG; 2020

[22] Brown CA. The Walls Manual of Emergency Airway Management. Sixth ed. NY: Lippincott Williams & Wilkins; 2023

[23] Díaz-Jimenez JP, Rodriguez AN. Interventions in Pulmonary Medicine. 2nd ed. NY: Springer International Publishing; 2018. DOI: 10.1007/978-3-319-58036-4

[24] Martinot A, Closset M, Marquette CH, et al. Indications for flexible versus rigid bronchoscopy in children with suspected foreign-body aspiration. American Journal of Respiratory and Critical Care Medicine. 1997;**155**(5):1676-1679. DOI: 10.1164/ajrccm.155.5.9154875

[25] Han LL, Meng C, Zhang ZX, et al. Clinical analysis of bronchoscope diagnosis and treatment for airway foreign body removal in pediatric patients. Italian Journal of Pediatrics. 2022;**48**:159. DOI: 10.1186/s13052-022-01347-x

[26] Chantzaras AP, Panagiotou P, Karageorgos S, Douros K. A systematic review of using flexible bronchoscopy to remove foreign bodies from paediatric patients. Acta Paediatrica. 2022;**111**(7):1301-1312. DOI: 10.1111/apa.16351

[27] Ikeda S, Yanai N, Ishikawa S. Flexible bronchofiberscope. The Keio Journal of Medicine. 1968;**17**(1):1-16. DOI: 10.2302/kjm.17.1

[28] Mise K, Jurcev Savicevic A, Pavlov N, Jankovic S. Removal of tracheobronchial foreign bodies in adults using flexible bronchoscopy: Experience 1995-2006. Surgical Endoscopy. 2009;**23**(6):1360-1364. DOI: 10.1007/s00464-008-0181-9

[29] Sehgal IS, Dhooria S, Ram B, et al. Foreign body inhalation in the adult population: Experience of 25,998 bronchoscopies and systematic review of the literature. Respiratory Care. 2015;**60**(10):1438-1448. DOI: 10.4187/respcare.03976

[30] Swanson KL. Airway foreign bodies: what's new? Seminars in Respiratory and Critical Care Medicine. 2004;**25**(4):405-411. DOI: 10.1055/s-2004-832713

[31] Mehta AC, Albert LR. Extraction of airway FB in adults. Journal of Bronchology. 2001;**8**(2):123-131

[32] Freiman MA, McMurray JS. Unique presentation of a bronchial foreign body in an asymptomatic child. The Annals of Otology, Rhinology, and Laryngology. 2001;**110**(6):495-497. DOI: 10.1177/000348940111000601

[33] Varshney R, Zawawi F, Shapiro A, Lacroix Y. Use of an endoscopic urology basket to remove bronchial foreign body in the pediatric population. International Journal of Pediatric Otorhinolaryngology. 2014;**78**(4):687-689. DOI: 10.1016/j.ijporl.2014.01.016

[34] Ichimura H, Maeda M, Kikuchi S, et al. Endobronchial dental prosthesis retrieval by a snare technique using a flexible bronchoscope and fluoroscopy: Two case reports and technical tips. Respiratory Medicine Case Reports. 2016;**19**:187-189. Published 2016 Oct 18. DOI: 10.1016/j.rmcr.2016.10.013

[35] Schmidt LH, Schulze AB, Goerlich D, et al. Blood clot removal by cryoextraction in critically ill patients with pulmonary hemorrhage. Journal of Thoracic Disease. 2019;**11**(10):4319-4327. DOI: 10.21037/jtd.2019.09.46

[36] Saito H, Saka H, Sakai S, Shimokata K. Removal of broken fragment of biopsy forceps with magnetic extractor. Chest. 1989;**95**(3):700-701. DOI: 10.1378/chest.95.3.700

[37] Mayr J, Dittrich S, Triebl K. A new method for removal of metallic-ferromagnetic foreign bodies from the tracheobronchial tree. Pediatric Surgery International. 1997;**12**(5-6):461-462. DOI: 10.1007/BF01076970

[38] Boelcskei PL, Wagner M, Lessnau KK. Laser-assisted removal of a foreign body in the bronchial system of an infant. Lasers in Surgery and Medicine. 1995;**17**(4):375-377. DOI: 10.1002/lsm.1900170407

[39] Fruchter O, Fox BD, Raviv Y, Kramer MR. Laser-assisted removal of aspirated thumbtacks by flexible bronchoscopy. Diagnostic and Therapeutic Endoscopy. 2010;**2010**:598760. DOI: 10.1155/2010/598760

[40] Debeljak A, Sorli J, Music E, Kecelj P. Bronchoscopic removal of foreign bodies in adults: Experience with 62 patients from 1974-1998. The European Respiratory Journal. 1999;**14**(4):792-795. DOI: 10.1034/j.1399-3003.1999.14d11.x

[41] Banerjee A, Rao KS, Khanna SK, et al. Laryngo-tracheo-bronchial foreign bodies in children. The Journal of Laryngology and Otology. 1988;**102**(11):1029-1032. DOI: 10.1017/s0022215100107170

[42] Bolliger CT. "Interventionelle Bronchoskopie" [interventional bronchoscopy]. Praxis. 1994;**83**(49):1378-1382

[43] Powers KF, Reese AD, Carr MM. Pediatric bronchoscopy for airway foreign bodies in the ACS NSQIP-P: Morbidity and mortality 2014-2019. The

Laryngoscope. 2023;**133**(3):689-693. DOI: 10.1002/lary.30170

[44] Ng J, Kim S, Chang B, et al. Clinical features and treatment outcomes of airway foreign body aspiration in adults. Journal of Thoracic Disease. 2019;**11**(3):1056-1064. DOI: 10.21037/jtd.2018.12.130

[45] Killian G. Father of bronchoscopy. Archives of Otolaryngology (1960), vol. 82, no. 6, 1965, pp. 656-659

[46] Higashi K, Takeshita J, Terasaki H, et al. A case of acute airway obstruction with sharp sawdust particles, successfully treated by extracorporeal lung assist. Kokyū to junkan. 1989;**37**(3):329-333

[47] Mellema JD, Bratton SL, Inglis A Jr, Morray JP. Use of cardiopulmonary bypass during bronchoscopy following sand aspiration. A case report. Chest. 1995;**108**(4):1176-1177. DOI: 10.1378/chest.108.4.1176

[48] Brown KL, Shefler A, Cohen G, DeMunter C, Pigott N, Goldman AP. Near-fatal grape aspiration with complicating acute lung injury successfully treated with extracorporeal membrane oxygenation. Pediatric Critical Care Medicine. 2003;**4**(2):243-245. DOI: 10.1097/01.PCC.0000059332.48377.7A

[49] Fernandez-Trujillo L, López-Castilla V, Morales EI, Zúñiga-Restrepo V, Bautista DF. Unsuspected foreign-body aspiration in adult patient with status asthmaticus: Case report. Annals of Medicine and Surgery (Lond). 2020;**56**: 1-4. Published 2020 Jun 8. DOI: 10.1016/j.amsu.2020.05.026

[50] Holliday T, Jackson A. Emergency use of extracorporeal membrane oxygenation for a foreign body obstructing the airway. Critical Care and Resuscitation. 2010;**12**(4):273-275

[51] Iwahashi H, Yuri K, Nosé Y. Development of the oxygenator: Past, present, and future. Journal of Artificial Organs. 2004;**7**(3):111-120. DOI: 10.1007/s10047-004-0268-6

[52] Hill JD, O'Brien TG, Murray JJ, et al. Prolonged extracorporeal oxygenation for acute post-traumatic respiratory failure (shock-lung syndrome). Use of the Bramson membrane lung. The New England Journal of Medicine. 1972;**286**(12):629-634. DOI: 10.1056/NEJM197203232861204

[53] Gropper M. Miller's Anesthesia. Elsevier; 2020

[54] Ignacio RC Jr, Falcone RA Jr, Brown RL. A case report of severe tracheal obstruction requiring extracorporeal membrane oxygenation. Journal of Pediatric Surgery. 2006;**41**(10):E1-E4. DOI: 10.1016/j.jpedsurg.2006.06.021

[55] Anton-Martin P, Bhattarai P, Rycus P, Raman L, Potera R. The use of extracorporeal membrane oxygenation in life-threatening foreign body aspiration: Case series, review of extracorporeal life support organization registry data, and systematic literature review. The Journal of Emergency Medicine. 2019;**56**(5):523-529. DOI: 10.1016/j.jemermed.2019.01.036

[56] Isherwood J, Firmin R. Late presentation of foreign body aspiration requiring extracorporeal membrane oxygenation support for surgical management. Interactive Cardiovascular and Thoracic Surgery. 2011;**12**(4):631-632. DOI: 10.1510/icvts.2010.249516

[57] Park AH, Tunkel DE, Park E, Barnhart D, Liu E, Lee J, et al.

Management of complicated airway foreign body aspiration using extracorporeal membrane oxygenation (ECMO). International Journal of Pediatric Otorhinolaryngology. 2014;**78**(12):2319-2321. DOI: 10.1016/j.ijporl.2014.10.021

[58] Razafimanjato NNM, Tsiambanizafy GO, Ravelomihary TDN, Rakotovao HJL, Hunald FA. Successful surgical repair of a sternum cleft using composite mesh: A case report and new technical note. African Journal of Thoracic and Critical Care Medicine. 2021;**27**(2):66-69. DOI: 10.7196/AJTCCM.2021.v27i2.103. Published 2021 Jun 23

[59] Razafimanjato NNM, Ralaivao RA, Ravelomihary TDN, Hunald FA, Rakotovao JLH. Pneumonectomy in a child due to belated diagnosis of foreign body aspiration: A case report. Journal of Medical Case Reports. 2021;**15**(1):533. Published 2021 Oct 20. DOI: 10.1186/s13256-021-03015-w

[60] Hrrmann D, Volmerig J, Wolf R, et al. Unterlappenektomie acht Jahre nach aspiration einer Pinnnadel [lobectomy of right lower lobe eight years after foreign body aspiration]. Pneumologie. 2019;**73**(4):240-243. DOI: 10.1055/a-0830-1524

Chapter 5

Foreign Bodies in Lower Airways in Children 1–3 Years Old

Melpomeni Bizhga

Abstract

The common symptoms of foreign body aspiration (FBA) include coughing, wheezing, choking, and respiratory distress. Physical examination may reveal abnormal respiratory sounds, such as wheezing or stridor, as well as signs of respiratory distress, such as increased respiratory rate, retractions, and nasal flaring. A chest X-ray is often the initial imaging modality used to evaluate foreign body aspiration. Bronchoscopy is considered the gold standard for both diagnosis and removal of foreign bodies in the airways. The diagnosis of foreign body aspiration in children aged 1–3 years requires a comprehensive approach that includes clinical evaluation, radiological imaging, and bronchoscopy. If the foreign body (FB) is causing significant airway obstruction, respiratory distress, or if it is not spontaneously expelled, a prompt removal of the foreign body is necessary. The most immediate and significant complication of foreign body aspiration is airway obstruction. In some cases, foreign body aspiration can lead to long-term complications, such as chronic suppurative lung disease (CSLD) or bronchiectasis. Foreign body aspiration in children can have a significant psychological impact on parents and caregivers. It is important for healthcare providers to be aware of these potential complications associated with flexible bronchoscopy in foreign bodies in children. Careful patient selection, expertise in the procedure, and appropriate monitoring can help minimize these risks.

Keywords: children, foreign body, lower airways, bronchoscopy, management

1. Introduction

Children from 1 to three years old are at greater risk of aspiration of foreign bodies in lower airways. This paper addresses clinicians to understand the physiopathology of aspiration, clinical signs, possible complications, and management of such a case.

2. Etiology and predisposing factors of foreign body aspiration

The clinical presentation of foreign body aspiration in children aged 1–3 years can vary depending on the type, size, and location of the foreign body. Common symptoms include coughing, wheezing, choking, and respiratory distress. However, it is important to note that the presentation can be nonspecific, leading to delayed diagnosis and potential complications.

Children from 1 to 3 years old have difficulties in coordinating breathing and swallowing.

Gag reflexes, cough, and glottic closure against chocking may not be fully developed from birth.

Children with development delays are at higher risk of aspiration in general and from aspiration of foreign bodies in airways especially. Children have smaller airways and even small changes in airway radius lead to much greater changes in airflow, decreasing dramatically airflow in airway (Flow = $1/R^4$) [1].

In an infant, the larynx is at a higher position and nearer to the base of the tongue, leading to more possible aspiration. Aspiration happens usually with organic materials, such as peanuts, nuts, seeds, or small pieces of toys, and at the same time children cry or laugh or run to escape the removal of the object from the mouth.

Secretion of mucus and edema of the bronchial mucosa can lead to further obstruction.

A study by Baharloo et al. [2] examined the clinical features of foreign body aspiration in children. They found that coughing was the most common symptom, present in 85.5% of cases, followed by wheezing (53.9%) and choking (39.2%). These findings highlight the importance of considering foreign body aspiration in the differential diagnosis of children presenting with respiratory symptoms.

Choking and asphyxia may happen as a first sign. This can be witnessed by caretakers and forgotten later on.

After penetration syndrome (when the foreign body bypasses subglottis) and choking seem to have already passed, the child may experience symptoms such as cough, stridor, or wheeze or may have minor symptoms, especially when the foreign body is lodged to one of the main bronchi.

This episode may be forgotten by caregivers or recalled when asked later.

Children may present at the clinician's office complaining of cough, fever, wheeze, etc. When the diagnosis is delayed, they may present with grave complications such as atelectasis, emphysema, pneumothorax, bronchiectasis, and chronic suppurative lung disease.

3. Fiz pathology of a foreign body in bronchus

Depending not only on the bronchus size and foreign body size, but also on the fact that usually foreign bodies in lower airways are usually vegetal and can raise their size due to humidity, they can impact aeration on the affected lung or bronchus in different ways:

1. When it does not affect either inspiration or expiration (on the first day of inspiration, a small foreign body): bypass valve, clinically and X-rays normal

2. When it does affect the expiration, but does not affect inspiration (edema of the bronchial wall, secretions from inflammation), check the valve mechanism

3. When it does affect the inspiration (a complete obstruction of the bronchus due to swelling of the vegetal foreign body), the residual air is absorbed gradually, which blocks the valve mechanism [3].

4. Diagnostic approach for foreign body aspiration

The clinical evaluation begins with a thorough history and physical examination. The healthcare provider will inquire about the child's symptoms, including coughing, wheezing, choking episodes, and any witnessed events of foreign body ingestion. The presence of risk factors, such as exposure to small objects or inadequate supervision, should also be assessed.

Physical examination may reveal abnormal respiratory sounds, such as wheezing or stridor, as well as signs of respiratory distress, such as increased respiratory rate, retractions, and nasal flaring. Cyanosis or other signs of inadequate oxygenation should also be assessed.

4.1 Radiological imaging

Chest X-ray: A chest X-ray is often the initial imaging modality used to evaluate foreign body aspiration. It is mandatory for all cases/suspected cases and can help to localize it through evaluating asymmetry, air trapping, mediastinal shift, and atelectasis. It is also important to differentiate other cases of respiratory distress not related to FBA.

In older children who can cooperate, inspiratory/expiratory films are more helpful. During expiratory films, mediastinal shifts are more obvious.

However, it is important to note that chest X-rays may not always detect radiolucent objects or early signs of aspiration. In one study [4] of 265 children with foreign bodies in airways, 110 of them had normal plain chest by the time they had bronchoscopy.

Only 10% of the foreign bodies on airways are radio opaque.

Chest radiographs may be normal in 17% of the foreign bodies in airways shown later on.

Pneumothorax or pneumomediastinum is found rarely. Their presence is dedicated to emphysema and flow through the fascia. When foreign bodies (FBs) (vegetal materials) carry germs, inflammation and infection can lead to pyopneumothoraxis.

4.2 Computed tomography (CT) scan

In stable children, CT and virtual bronchoscopy are more useful compared to plain X-ray Adaletli et al. [5]. In cases where the chest X-ray is inconclusive or there is a high suspicion of foreign body aspiration, a computed tomography (CT) scan may be performed. CT scans provide more detailed images of the airways and can help identify smaller or radiolucent foreign bodies. It is especially useful in cases where there is a concern for complications or when bronchoscopy is planned.

4.3 Bronchoscopy

Bronchoscopy is considered the gold standard for both diagnosis and removal of foreign bodies in the airways. It involves inserting a flexible or rigid bronchoscope through the mouth or nose to visualize the airways and remove the foreign body if present. Bronchoscopy allows direct visualization of the airways, identification of the foreign body's location, and assessment of any airway- associated injury or inflammation.

In some cases, bronchoscopy may be performed urgently if there is a complete airway obstruction or significant respiratory distress. In other cases, it may be performed electively after initial evaluation and imaging. The timing and approach to bronchoscopy depend on the clinical presentation, radiological findings, and the expertise available in the healthcare setting.

The diagnosis of foreign body aspiration in children aged 1–3 years requires a comprehensive approach that includes clinical evaluation, radiological imaging, and bronchoscopy. Chest X-rays are commonly used as an initial diagnostic tool, but they may not always detect radiolucent objects or early signs of aspiration. There are studies that show that X-rays on the first 24 hours of a foreign body aspiration are normal.

It requires a high index of suspicion from the clinician when evaluating a child from 1 to 3 years old with cough and indirect signs in X-rays.

Persistent atelectasis, hyperventilation of a lobe, or the lung accompanied by dull sounds on auscultation might rise the suspicion of a foreign body aspiration lodged on lower airways.

A study by E. Svedström et al. [6] in an analysis of a radiograph of 83 consecutive patients, in which the prevalence of FB aspiration was 41%, the diagnostic accuracy was 67%, sensitivity 68% and specificity 67%. Therefore, a negative chest X-ray does not rule out foreign body aspiration, and further evaluation is necessary.

When there is a history of choking and there are clinical signs as cough, wheeze, and/or indirect radiological signs such as: hyperventilated lung or lobe, atelectasis, or persistent pneumonia, the diagnosis of confirmation/exclusion of a foreign body in airways should be made.

Clinical signs that show a possible foreign body in trachea should indicate prompt rigid bronchoscopy. Persistent pneumonia or radiological signs of emphysema of the lobe or the lung may first require a flexible bronchoscopy.

5. Management of foreign body aspiration

Foreign body aspiration in children requires prompt and appropriate management to ensure the child's safety and prevent complications. The management approach involves a combination of supportive care, removal of the foreign body, and follow-up care.

5.1 Supportive care

In cases of partial airway obstruction or mild symptoms, supportive care may be sufficient. This includes closely monitoring the child's respiratory status, providing reassurance, and ensuring a calm environment. Encouraging the child to cough and maintaining an upright position can help facilitate the spontaneous expulsion of the foreign body.

In infants, back slap with the head down, chest thrust, or a combination of both is encouraged when asphyxia happens after witnessing the episode of choking.

In older children, Heimlich maneuver is more effective.

5.2 Removal of the foreign body

If the foreign body is causing significant airway obstruction, respiratory distress, or if it is not spontaneously expelled, a prompt removal is necessary. The primary method of removal is through bronchoscopy, which allows direct visualization and retrieval of the foreign body.

Bronchoscopy can be performed using a flexible or a rigid bronchoscope, depending on the availability and expertise of the healthcare setting. The procedure is typically performed under general anesthesia to ensure the child's comfort and safety.

During bronchoscopy, the foreign body is located and removed using various instruments, such as forceps or suction catheters.

The management of foreign body aspiration in children aged 1–3 years involves ensuring a patent airway, providing appropriate oxygenation, and removing the foreign body. Bronchoscopy is considered the gold standard for both diagnosis and removal of foreign bodies.

A study by Cheng et al. [7] assessed the outcomes of bronchoscopic removal of foreign bodies in children. They reported a success rate of 97.6% and a low complication rate. This study emphasizes the importance of prompt bronchoscopy intervention for optimal management of foreign body aspiration.

Both rigid bronchoscopy and flexible bronchoscopy are used to remove a foreign body from lower airways.

Despite a lot of studies showing the efficacy of flexible bronchoscopy on removal of foreign bodies in airways, interventionists should always have a backup of rigid bronchoscopy.

Rigid bronchoscopy requires general anesthesia, but allows control of the airways at the same time, as the instrument is advanced to remove the foreign body in a safe way, also facilitating mucus plugging aspiration at the same time and installation of saline or mucolytics in the collapsed area.

If a foreign body is surrounded by granulation tissue, a balloon catheter may be used in order to ensure removal of a round object under the granulation. Prevention of disintegration of vegetal foreign bodies is important, in order to prevent smaller parts obstructing more peripheral airways.

On rare circumstances, when the foreign body gets stuck on the subglottic area during removal (monkey trap), it should be moved downward where the trachea is wider and allows oxygenation. Emergency tracheostomy may be required. Rigid bronchoscopy has the advantage of proper oxygenation during the procedure and the removal can take more time. Another advantage is bypassing the risk of the foreign body getting stuck on subglottic area that may lead to asphyxia when removal is effectuated with a flexible bronchoscope.

Flexible bronchoscopy is increasingly used for the removal of the foreign body. In a study on more than 1000 children, foreign bodies were successfully removed in 90% of them. Flexible bronchoscopy is recommended especially in distant foreign bodies in airways and for upper lobe lodged foreign bodies.

Management of complications from a long-standing foreign body as bronchiectasis may require lobectomy.

6. Anesthesia regime for flexible bronchoscopy and for rigid bronchoscopy

For flexible bronchoscopy, spontaneous breathing is possible with the use of propofol, propofol plus sevoflurane, and midazolam as anxiolytic. On the other hand, for rigid bronchoscopy paralysis is indicated rather than spontaneous ventilation. There is a lack of consensus about the regime Fidkowski et al. [8]. As regards foreign bodies in a child, any procedure such as positive end-expiratory pressure (PEEP) is recommended in order to reinflate the parts of the collapsed lung and adrenaline 1:1000 is applied locally in minor bleedings after the removal.

Antibiotics are used for several days after removal. Steroids are used for short courses to decrease edema of the airways.

All other bronchi are checked to rule out any other foreign body lodged there.

6.1 Follow-up care

After successful removal of the foreign body, a close follow-up care is essential. The child should be monitored for any signs of complications, such as persistent respiratory symptoms, recurrent infections, or airway injury. Follow-up visits with the healthcare provider may be scheduled to assess the child's respiratory status and ensure proper healing.

6.2 Prevention

Prevention is crucial in reducing the risk of foreign body aspiration in children. Parents and caregivers should be educated about potential choking hazards and the importance of providing a safe environment for the child. This includes keeping small objects out of reach, ensuring proper supervision during playtime and meals, and promoting age-appropriate toy selection.

In summary, the management of foreign body aspiration in children involves supportive care, prompt removal of the foreign body through bronchoscopy, and close follow-up care. Prevention plays a vital role in reducing the risk of aspiration and should be emphasized to parents and caregivers.

7. Complications and prognosis of foreign body aspiration

Foreign body aspiration in children can lead to various complications, some of which can be serious and potentially life-threatening. The prognosis of foreign body aspiration depends on several factors, including the type and location of the foreign body, the duration of the obstruction, and the promptness of medical intervention.

7.1 Complications

1. Airway obstruction: The most immediate and significant complication of foreign body aspiration is airway obstruction. This can cause respiratory distress, cyanosis, and even respiratory arrest, if not promptly addressed. Complete obstruction requires urgent intervention to restore the airway and ensure adequate oxygenation.

2. Respiratory infections: Aspiration of a foreign body can lead to respiratory infections, such as pneumonia or bronchitis. The presence of a foreign body in the airways can obstruct normal airflow, trap bacteria, and cause inflammation, increasing the risk of infection. Prompt removal of the foreign body and appropriate antibiotic therapy are essential to prevent or treat respiratory infections.

3. Airway injury: The presence of a foreign body in the airways can cause injury to the surrounding tissues. This can result in inflammation, edema, and even ulceration or perforation of the airway walls. Airway injury may require additional interventions, such as medication to reduce inflammation or surgical repair, depending on the severity.

4. Long-term complications: In some cases, foreign body aspiration can lead to long-term complications, such as chronic suppurative lung disease or bronchiectasis. These conditions can result from recurrent respiratory infections,

persistent inflammation, or damage to the airway structures. Close follow-up care and appropriate management are important to monitor and address any potential long-term complications.

7.2 Prognosis

The prognosis of foreign body aspiration depends on several factors. Prompt recognition and intervention are crucial in preventing complications and improving outcomes. The prognosis is generally favorable when the foreign body is promptly removed and there are no significant complications.

However, the prognosis may be influenced by factors such as the type and size of the foreign body, the duration of the obstruction, the presence of associated injuries or infections, and the child's overall health. In some cases, the prognosis may be less favorable if there are significant complications or delays in diagnosis and treatment.

It is important to note that each case is unique, and the prognosis should be discussed with the healthcare provider based on the specific circumstances.

8. Case study of a foreign body in airways

Nursing diagnosis (ND), female, 2 years old, 1 week with fever, admitted to hospital as having pneumonia. Child was alert, no respiratory distress, sat O2 96%, respiratory frequency (FR) 36/min, and cardiac rate (FK) 106/min.

Decreased breath sounds on the left side. Some bronchial rale on the right side.

Blood workup normal. X-ray is shown (**Figure 1**):

After evaluation of X-rays, the caregivers were asked about the possibility of a foreign body aspiration. They denied at first and then admitted that 2 weeks ago all the family had consumed sunflower seeds and the child as well.

Flexible bronchoscopy was performed and a sunflower seed was found on the end of left main bronchus (**Figures 2** and **3**).

Removal of the foreign body was made possible by rigid bronchoscopy. Treatment after removal included antibiotics, short-acting corticosteroids (**Figure 4**).

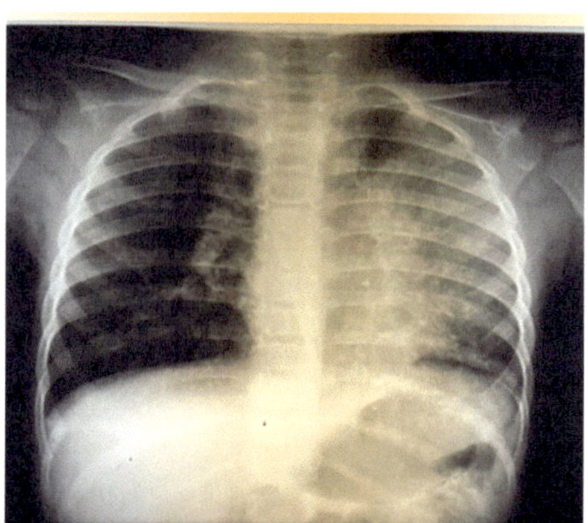

Figure 1.
Atelectasis of the left lung. Mediastinal shift to the left side.

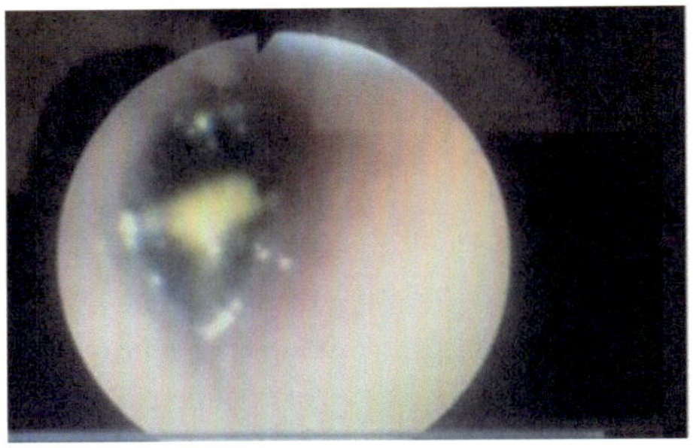

Figure 2.
Flexible bronchoscopic view of the foreign body on lower left bronchus.

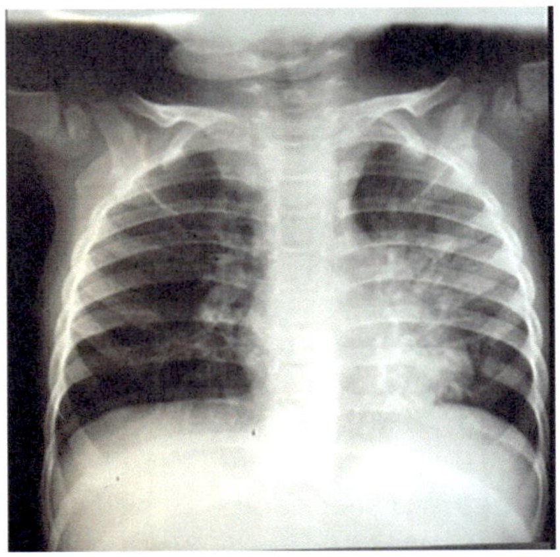

Figure 3.
X-rays after removal of the foreign body (FB). RI expansion of the reopening of lung. Some left perihilar consolidation.

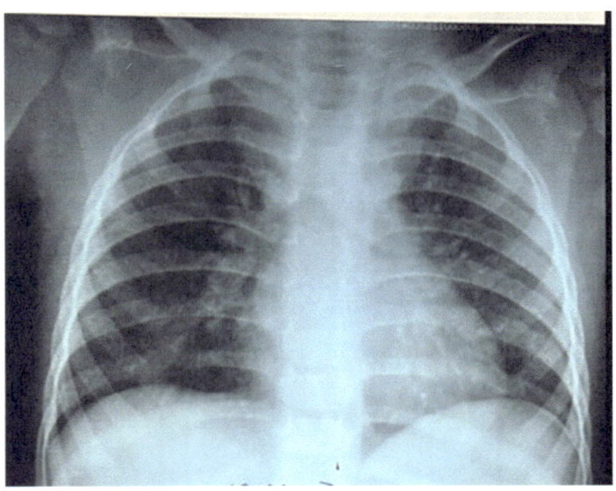

Figure 4.
X-rays after 5 days of treatment with antibiotics and steroids. Normal findings.

9. Psychological impact of foreign body aspiration on parents and caregivers

Foreign body aspiration in children can have a significant psychological impact on parents and caregivers. The experience of witnessing a child choking or struggling to breathe can be traumatic and distressing. The psychological impact can vary from mild anxiety and worry to more severe emotional distress and post-traumatic stress symptoms.

1. Acute stress reaction: Parents and caregivers may experience acute stress reactions immediately following the incident. This can include symptoms, such as fear, helplessness, guilt, and intrusive thoughts or nightmares about the event. They may also experience physical symptoms like increased heart rate, sweating, or difficulty sleeping.

2. Anxiety and worry: After the incident, parents and caregivers may develop heightened anxiety and worry about their child's safety and well-being. They may become overly cautious or hypervigilant, constantly monitoring the child's activities and surroundings to prevent any potential harm. This anxiety can persist, even after the foreign body has been successfully removed.

3. Guilt and self-blame: Parents and caregivers may experience feelings of guilt and self-blame, questioning their own actions or supervision during the incident. They may blame themselves for not preventing the aspiration or for not recognizing the signs earlier. It is important to reassure parents and caregivers that foreign body aspiration can occur, even with the best supervision and that seeking prompt medical attention is crucial.

4. Post-traumatic stress disorder (PTSD): In some cases, parents and caregivers may develop symptoms of post-traumatic stress disorder (PTSD). This can include flashbacks, nightmares, avoidance of reminders of the event, and persistent anxiety or hypervigilance. If these symptoms persist and significantly impact daily functioning, it is important to seek professional help.

5. Support and coping strategies: It is crucial to provide support and resources to parents and caregivers to help them cope with the psychological impact of foreign body aspiration. This can include offering reassurance, providing accurate information about the incident and its management, and connecting them with support groups or counseling services. Encouraging self-care and stress management techniques can also be beneficial.

It is important to recognize that the psychological impact can vary from person to person, and individuals may have different coping mechanisms. Providing a supportive and understanding environment can help parents and caregivers navigate through their emotions and seek appropriate help if needed.

10. Education and awareness for foreign bodies

Education and awareness about foreign bodies are essential in preventing incidents of aspiration, especially in children. By providing information and promoting safety measures, we can help reduce the risk of foreign body aspiration and its associated complications. Here are some key aspects of education and awareness for foreign bodies:

1. Parent and caregiver education: Parents and caregivers should be educated about the common objects that pose a risk for aspiration, such as small toys, coins, buttons, and food items. They should be aware of the signs and symptoms of foreign body aspiration, including coughing, choking, wheezing, and difficulty in breathing. Providing information on proper supervision and age-appropriate toys can also help prevent incidents.

2. Safe eating practices: Educating parents and caregivers about safe eating practices is crucial in preventing food-related foreign body aspiration. This includes cutting food into appropriate sizes for children, encouraging them to chew food thoroughly, and avoiding giving young children foods that are hard, small, or sticky. Emphasizing the importance of sitting down and eating slowly can also reduce the risk of choking.

3. First aid training: Basic first aid training can be valuable in emergency situations. Parents, caregivers, and even older children should be educated on how to perform the Heimlich maneuver or back blows to relieve airway obstruction in case of choking. This knowledge can help save lives during critical moments before medical professionals arrive [9].

4. Public awareness campaigns: Public awareness campaigns can play a significant role in educating the general population about the risks and prevention of foreign body aspiration. These campaigns can utilize various platforms, such as social media, television, and community events, to reach a wide audience. Providing clear and concise information, along with practical tips, can help raise awareness and encourage proactive measures.

5. Healthcare provider education: Healthcare providers, including pediatricians, nurses, and emergency personnel, should receive education and training on the recognition and management of foreign body aspiration. They should be familiar with the appropriate diagnostic tools, such as X-rays or bronchoscopy, and the recommended interventions for different scenarios. Continuous education and updates on guidelines can ensure that healthcare providers are equipped to handle these cases effectively.

6. Collaboration with schools and childcare centers: Collaboration with schools and childcare centers is crucial in promoting safety and awareness. Educators and staff should be trained in recognizing signs of foreign body aspiration and responding appropriately. Creating a safe environment with age-appropriate toys and regular inspections of play areas can also minimize the risk of incidents.

By implementing comprehensive education and awareness programs, we can empower individuals, families, and communities to take proactive measures in preventing foreign body aspiration. This can ultimately reduce the number of incidents and improve the overall safety and well-being of children.

11. Conclusions on foreign bodies in children

Foreign body aspiration in children is a serious concern that requires attention and proactive measures to prevent and manage. Here are some key conclusions regarding foreign bodies in children:

1. Prevention is key: Education, awareness, and proactive measures are crucial in preventing incidents of foreign body aspiration in children. By providing information to parents, caregivers, and the general public about the common objects that pose a risk, safe eating practices, and first aid techniques, we can reduce the occurrence of these incidents.

2. Supervision and age-appropriate toys: Proper supervision is essential in ensuring the safety of children, especially during playtime and mealtime. Parents and caregivers should be vigilant and provide age-appropriate toys and foods to minimize the risk of choking or aspiration.

3. Prompt recognition and response: Recognizing the signs and symptoms of foreign body aspiration is vital for prompt intervention. Parents, caregivers, and healthcare providers should be aware of the common symptoms, such as coughing, choking, wheezing, and difficulty in breathing. Knowing how to perform basic first aid techniques, such as the Heimlich maneuver, can be life-saving in emergency situations.

4. Collaboration and education: Collaboration between healthcare providers, schools, childcare centers, and parents is essential in promoting safety and awareness. Healthcare providers should receive education and training on the recognition and management of foreign body aspiration, while schools and childcare centers should implement safety measures and educate staff and parents about prevention.

5. Psychological impact: Foreign body aspiration can have a significant psychological impact on parents and caregivers. It is important to provide support, reassurance, and resources to help them cope with the emotional aftermath of such incidents.

6. Continuous improvement: Ongoing research, education, and awareness campaigns are necessary to continuously improve our understanding and prevention strategies for foreign body aspiration in children. By staying updated with the latest guidelines and sharing knowledge, we can work toward reducing the incidence and impact of these incidents.

In conclusion, foreign body aspiration in children is a preventable and manageable condition. By focusing on prevention, prompt recognition, and collaboration, we can create a safer environment for children and reduce the occurrence of these incidents. Additionally, addressing the psychological impact on parents and caregivers is crucial for their well-being. With continuous improvement and education, we can strive to minimize the risks associated with foreign body aspiration and ensure the safety and health of children.

12. Complications of flexible bronchoscopy in foreign bodies in children—Literature review

Flexible bronchoscopy is a valuable diagnostic and therapeutic tool for the management of foreign bodies in the lower airways of children. While it is generally considered safe and effective, there are potential complications that healthcare providers should be aware of. Here is a literature review of the complications associated with flexible bronchoscopy in foreign bodies in children:

Complications of foreign body aspiration are;

1. Physiological, due to hypoxemia, with or without hypercapnia.

2. Mechanical, as is epistaxis, hemoptysis, pneumothorax, or post subglottic edema.

3. Infectious (bacteriological complications).

4. Anesthetic, when most life-threatening adverse events involve: overdose, inadequate monitoring, or inappropriate sedation

5. Post bronchoalveolar lavage (BAL) fever

J de Blic et al. [10] described in a study with 1328 procedures, 1153 children, who underwent diagnostic procedures of flexible bronchoscopy, presented major complications such as important desaturation (oxygen saturation value (Sat O2) <90%), 21 children (1,6%) had all procedures done, 6 children (0,6%) suffered from laryngospasm, and one patient (0,1%) presented difficulty due to pneumothorax.

Six children (0,5%) presented minor complications such as epistaxis, whereas 15 children (1,1%) presented isolated desaturation.

Ninety-one patients (6,9%) presented overall complications (at least one).

The majority of procedures were performed under conscious sedation (93%), and only 7% of procedures were performed under deep sedation.

Complications of flexible bronchoscopy are:

1. Bleeding: Several studies have reported bleeding as a potential complication of flexible bronchoscopy in children. The incidence of bleeding varies, ranging from minor mucosal bleeding to more significant bleeding requiring intervention. Careful technique and expertise are necessary to minimize the risk of bleeding.

2. Airway injury: Airway injury, including mucosal abrasions, edema, or even perforation, can occur during the manipulation of the bronchoscope in the airways of children. The literature suggests that airway injury is more common in younger children due to the smaller size and more delicate airway structures. Proper training and experience are crucial to minimize the risk of airway injury.

3. Infection: The introduction of a foreign object (the bronchoscope) into the airways can increase the risk of infection. While rare, cases of airway infection following flexible bronchoscopy in children have been reported in the literature. Proper sterilization and disinfection techniques should be followed to minimize the risk of introducing bacteria or other pathogens into the airways.

4. Respiratory compromise: The presence of a foreign body in the lower airways can already cause partial or complete airway obstruction in children. During the removal procedure, there is a risk of dislodging the foreign body and causing further airway compromise. This can lead to respiratory distress or even respiratory arrest, requiring immediate intervention.

5. Anesthesia-related complications: Flexible bronchoscopy in children is often performed under sedation or general anesthesia. While generally safe, there are inherent risks associated with anesthesia, such as allergic reactions, respiratory depression, or cardiovascular complications. Proper patient selection, monitoring, and anesthesia management are crucial to minimize these risks.

6. Failure to remove the foreign body: The literature suggests that the success rate of foreign body removal using flexible bronchoscopy in children is generally high. However, in some cases, the removal may not be successful due to factors such as the size, shape, and location of the foreign body, as well as patient factors. In such cases, alternative methods, such as rigid bronchoscopy or surgical intervention, may be required.

It is important for healthcare providers to be aware of these potential complications associated with flexible bronchoscopy in foreign bodies in children. A careful patient selection, expertise in the procedure, and appropriate monitoring can help minimize these risks. Additionally, prompt recognition and management of complications are crucial for ensuring optimal outcomes.

Author details

Melpomeni Bizhga
University Hospital "Nene Tereza", Service of Specialties 1, Pediatrics, Tirane, Albania

*Address all correspondence to: melpomenibizhga@yahoo.com

References

[1] West JB. Respiratory Physiology: The Essentials. 7th ed. Lippincot Williams Wilkins; 2004. pp. 114-115

[2] Baharloo F, Veyckemans F, Francis C, et al. Tracheobronchial foreign bodies: Presentation and management in children and adults. Chest. 1999;**115**:1357-1362

[3] English GM. Disorders of the bronchi. Otolaryngology. 1992;**3**:43-47

[4] Zerrella J et al. Foreign body aspiration in children: Value of radiography and complications of bronchoscopy. Journal of Pediatric Surgery. 1998;**33**(11):1651-1654

[5] Adaletli I et al. Utilization of low dose multidetector Ct and virtual bronchoscopy in children with foreign body aspiration. Pediatric Radiology. 2007;**37**:33-40

[6] Svedström E, Puhakka H, Kero P. How accurate is chest radiography in the diagnosis of tracheobronchial foreign bodies in children? Pediatric Radiology. 1989;**19**:520-522

[7] Cheng W et al. Foreign body ingestion in children: Experience with 1265 cases. Journal of Pediatric Surgery. 1999;**34**(10):1472-1476

[8] Fidkowski CW et al. The anesthetic considerations of tracheobronchial foreign bodies in children: A literature review of 12979 cases. Anesthesia and Analgesia. 2010;**111**:1016-1025

[9] Nolan JP et al. Section 1, executive summary. Resuscitation. 2010;**81**(10):1219-1276

[10] de Blic J, Marchac V, Scheinmann P. Complications of flexible bronchoscopy in children: Prospective study of 1328 procedures. The European Respiratory Journal. 2002;**20**:1271

Section 3

Ear Foreign Body

Chapter 6

Foreign Body in the Ear

Jacky Munilson, Yan Edward and Emilia Nissa Khairani

Abstract

Foreign bodies are all objects that are not normally present in the human body. In the context of ear foreign bodies, the sophisticated structures of ear itself allow any materials that enter through the external auditory canal to become impacted. The prevalence of foreign bodies in the ear varies by gender and sex and depends on any other condition that may affect them. The clinical manifestation of foreign bodies in the ear may vary based on the material, location and duration of impaction. The removal of ear foreign bodies is performed using various kind of instrumentation and technique, considering how complex the removal is to be performed. Some complications may emerge either from the foreign bodies itself or the attempts of removal.

Keywords: *ear foreign* bodies, external auditory canal, impaction, instrumentation, removal

1. Introduction

Foreign bodies are all objects that come from inside or outside the body that are not normally present in the human body and can cause damage if not immediately medical intervention. Foreign bodies in the ear are commonly present in the emergency department worldwide. Children represent the majority of the population.

2. Anatomy of the ear

2.1 External ear

The external ear consists of the earlobe (auricle/pinna) and the ear canal (external auditory canal (EAC)). The pinna, apart from the lobules and the outer part of the internal acoustic canal, is formed by an arrangement of thin cartilage, which is then covered by skin to form the characteristic shape of the earlobe [1, 2]. Therefore, the earlobe also plays a role in cosmetics.

The movement of the earlobe is assisted by intrinsic and extrinsic muscles through the innervation of the facial nerve. The superficial temporal artery, which originates from branches of the external carotid artery, supplies the auricle anteriorly and from the posterior auricular artery toward the lateral helix [3–5].

External auditory canal is after the pinna, which then leads to the tympanic membrane. This pathway is formed by a combination of elastic cartilage on the 1/3 outer (lateral) and bone on the 2/3 inner (medial) so that a narrowing of the diameter is often found at the transition between cartilage and bone (isthmus). After passing through the isthmus, you will find a structure called the anterior recess [1–4]. If there are foreign objects in these parts, extraction will be difficult (see **Figure 1**). Apart from that, there are several other structures around the ear canal. At the anterior of the canal, the parotid gland and temporomandibular articulation are found. The posterior of ear canal is marked by the mastoid process [1, 4].

Ear canal which is a 24 mm long curved path leads to the tympanic membrane. The outer part curves upwards, downwards, then medially. Meanwhile, in the inside, the path turns downwards, straight, then medially. Therefore, it is necessary to modify the way the pinna is pulled upwards, backward, and laterally during a physical examination of the ear [2].

Similar to the earlobe, the 1/3 outer of the ear canal is also lined with skin and contains several glands, sebaceous and ceruminous. The skin in the ear canal is innervated by the auriculotemporal nerve and the auricular ramus of the vagus nerve. Lymph flow in the ear canal is directed toward the surrounding lymph nodes, in the cervical, parotid and mastoid areas [1]. Therefore, caution is needed in the management of foreign bodies because interventions such as pressure applied to the ear canal can stimulate the vagal reflex and cause the patient to vomit and cough [6].

2.2 Middle ear

2.2.1 Tympanic cavity

The tympanic cavity is an air cavity in the middle ear, in the pars petrosa of the temporal bone. This cavity contains the tympanic membrane, which connects to the auditory ossicles. The tympanic cavity communicates with the nasopharynx at the anterior and the mastoid antrum at the posterior. This space is lined with a mucous membrane and filled with air inside. Based on its location on the pars tensa of tympanic membrane, the space is divided into epitympanum, mesotympanum and hypotympanum [1–4].

The structure of the tympanic cavity is built by the roof, floor and anterior, posterior, lateral and medial walls. The roof is built by the structure of the tegmen tympani and the floor or base of the ear cavity is limited by the roof of the jugular bulb, which will become the sigmodeus and transverse sinuses. The walls of the

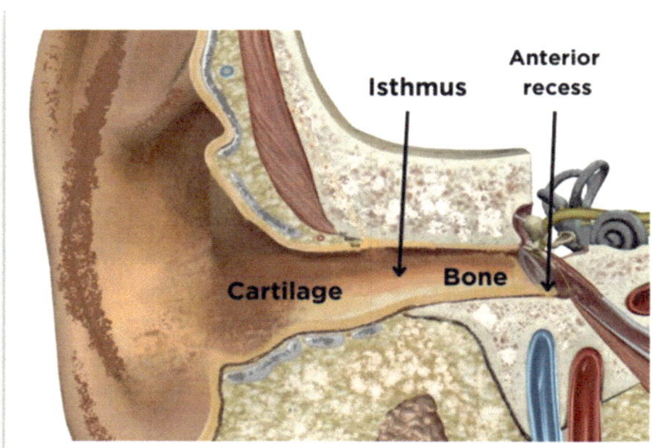

Figure 1.
Anatomy of the external ear.

tympanic cavity are formed by the tympanic membrane on the lateral side. The lateral wall is also formed by the epitympanum and hypotympanum bones. In the medial part, the lateral wall of the posterior cranial fossa or the lateral wall of the inner ear. On the medial wall, there is promontory, a protrusion originating from the first layer of the cochlea. The floor of the middle cranial fossa forms the superior wall so that the tympanic cavity can be separated from the internal carotid artery. On the posterior wall, you can find the aditus ad antrum along with the pyramid where the tendon of the stapedius muscle exits [3, 4]. Overall, the structures that make up the walls of the middle ear make the tympanic cavity a space with a narrower central portion.

2.2.2 Tympanic membrane

The tympanic membrane is a thin, round, fibrous membrane with a diameter of less than 1 centimeter and forms the lateral wall of the tympanic cavity. Laterally, the tympanic membrane forms a depression, which then becomes the top of the membrane. This peak is called the umbo and plays a role in producing the cone of light. This formation is caused by the attachment of the manubrium malei by the mucous membrane to the inner surface of the tympanic membrane [3, 4].

The tympanic membrane has three layers. The first layer is the skin layer (epidermis), the second layer is composed of fibrous and the third layer on the inside is the mucosa layer. The edge of the tympanic membrane thickens and is then divided into two parts by the anterior and posterior plica mallearis; pars tensa and pars flaccida (*Shrapnell's* membrane) [4]. The auriculotemporal nerve and the auricular ramus of the vagus nerve supply innervation to the outer surface of the tympanic membrane [3].

The tympanic membrane is 9-10 mm in height with a width of up to 8-9 mm. Meanwhile, the thickness of the tympanic membrane reaches 0.1 mm. The position of the tympanic membrane is tilted at 55 degrees to the external auditory canal. On otoscopic examination, several structures of the tympanic membrane and its surroundings can be seen, for example, the attic, manubrium malei, cone of light and several middle ear structures depicted on the tympanic membrane [1, 2].

2.2.3 Ossicle auditus

The auditory ossicles or auditory ossicles in the middle ear consist of three bones. These bones, in sequence from lateral to medial, are the malleus, incus and stapes. The ossicula auditus is also supported by several muscles and their innervation [3, 4].

The malleus or hammer bone is an auditory bone that is directly connected to the tympanic membrane and is also the largest bone among the other auditory bones. The length of the malleus reaches 8 mm. Its connection to the tympanic membrane is formed through the attachment of the lateral process. Other structures of the malleus consist of the head, column, manubrium and anterior process. The manubrium malei is the insertion of the tensor tympani muscle which is innervated by the trigeminal nerve of the mandibular division [1, 4]. The incus or anvil bone is the auditory bone after the malleus. The incus is connected to the malleus through its corpus in the head of the malei. Apart from that, the incus has two crus; the crus longum and the crus breve. During otoscope examination, the crus longum is often seen as a shadow on the tympanic membrane. Meanwhile, the crus breve protrudes and is attached to the posterior wall of the middle ear [4]. The stapes consist of the head, collar and base. At the neck of the stapes, the stapedius muscle inserts from its origin in the pyramid and is innervated by the facial nerve. Therefore, stapes vibrations can be dampened [3, 4].

2.2.4 Auditory tube

The auditory tube or eustachian tube is a canal that connects the nasopharynx to the middle ear so that the air pressure in the tympanic cavity and nasopharynx or the air pressure on both sides of the tympanic membrane remains balanced. The auditory tube is formed by cartilage in the anterior two-thirds (medial) and bone in the one-third posterior (lateral). The tensor tympani muscle originates above the bony posterior part. The part of the tube formed on the cartilage then enters the pharynx in a position above the superior pharyngeal constrictor muscle [3, 4].

The eustachian tube is tilted downwards at 45 degrees. The diameter of the eustachian tube is different in each section. In the bony part, the tube diameter reaches 3–6 mm. When it reaches the transition point to the cartilaginous part (isthmus), the diameter becomes narrower, about 1–2 mm [7].

2.2.5 Mastoid antrum

The antrum mastoid is an air-filled cavity with 9 mm height, 14 mm width and 7 mm depth. This cavity is at the top of the mastoid and contains air cells. The air cells are separated into various cell groups; zygomatic cells, tegmen cells, perisinus cells, retrofacial cells, perilabyrinth cells, perituba cells, tip cells, marginal cells and squamous cells [1].

The mastoid cavity has the shape of a three-sided pyramid, which is sequentially formed by the middle cranial fossa, lateral posterior cranial fossa, subcutaneous bone in the posterior area of the auricle, and the aditus ad antrum as the roof, medial wall, lateral wall and anterior wall. Behind the tympanic cavity of the pars petrosa of temporal bone, there is the mastoid antrum, which is connected to the cavity via the aditus and is where the lateral semicircular canal protrudes. In this area, the facial nerve exits the temporal bone through the stylomastoid foramen [3, 4].

3. Epidemiology

Foreign bodies in the ear are commonly present in the emergency department worldwide. Children represent the majority of the population. There have been studies in countries worldwide reporting the epidemiology of foreign bodies. A retrospective study was conducted on pediatric patients aged under 16 years old, presenting to the ED of Women's and Children's Hospital in Singapore for foreign bodies in the ear over 4 years from 2013 to 2017. The largest age group consisted of 53.7% of preschool children aged 0 to 6 years. The remainder included 40.6% of children aged 7 to 12 years and 5.7% above 12 years. The median age was 5.8. Male-to-female ratio of 1.6:1. The most common objects were organic materials including paper, cotton buds, tissue and erasers, followed by beads and stones, inorganic materials, as well as toys. There were cases involving insects and button batteries. More than half of the foreign bodies were found in the right ear, 37.8% in the left ear and 5.5% had bilateral involvement. Most foreign bodies were predominantly lodged in the external auditory canal and could be seen on direct visualization [8].

In older babies and toddlers, the development of the hand's grasping ability improves, allowing them to hold small objects and insert them into the ear canal. Apart from that, this can occur due to boredom, curiosity and a desire to imitate adults [9, 10].

Foreign body impaction in adults usually occurs as a result of cleaning or scratching the ear canal using various tools, such as cotton buds and matchsticks. In a retrospective review of 123 cases, ear foreign bodies were found in 11.4% of cases, all of which occurred in adults [11].

Apart from the pediatric population, people with mental disorders, hyperkinetic disorders and learning disorders also quite often insert foreign objects into the ear [8, 12]. People who experience physical abuse are also not spared. Therefore, a detailed history regarding the chronology of foreign bodies in patients needs to be carried out by a doctor [13, 14]. Most of the existing studies were conducted on the largest sample of right-handed users. The results showed that ear foreign bodies were more commonly found in right-handed users [14, 15].

4. Definition

Foreign bodies are all objects that come from inside or outside the body that are not normally present in the human body and can cause damage if you do not immediately get medical help. A variety of foreign bodies are found in the ear. Foreign bodies in the ear can be insects or parts of plants. In children, foreign bodies are often found in the form of beads, toys, erasers, green beans and batteries. Foreign bodies in adults include cotton buds, matches and insects [9, 16].

5. Classification of the foreign body

Organic materials were the most common type of foreign bodies in the ear, including paper, tissue fragments and cotton buds. Small inorganic objects such as beads and stones were the next most common foreign bodies. These objects are easily available in the household and are easy to be inserted into the ear by children due to unsepervision [8]. Another type of foreign body is live foreign bodies such as insects. Be aware of the type of foreign body will help us decide the most suitable method or technique and instruments that we will use to extract the foreign body. See **Figure 2** for various types of foreign bodies in the ear.

The patient's age typically determines the sort of foreign body. The incidence of foreign items is concentrated in two peak ages, which are 3–6 years and 17–18 years. Though the majority is male in general, women predominate in the 17–18 age range. This could be explained by the trend of teenage girls starting to wear jewelry more often, such as pierced ears or earrings [13]. Toy pieces such as marbles or toy gun bullets are frequently included in foreign body cases involving children under the age of 10. The kind of foreign object will become more associated with everyday actions as one gets older, such as cotton bud residue from self-picking. Additionally, because the EAC has a broader diameter in adult patients, the foreign body will typically be larger in size [9]. Other types that are most common in adults can be insects or earring parts.

5.1 Animate vs. non-animate

Living foreign bodies are usually insects, for example, flies, mosquitoes, grasshoppers, maggots, ticks and those that crawl, such as cockroaches, beetles or ants.

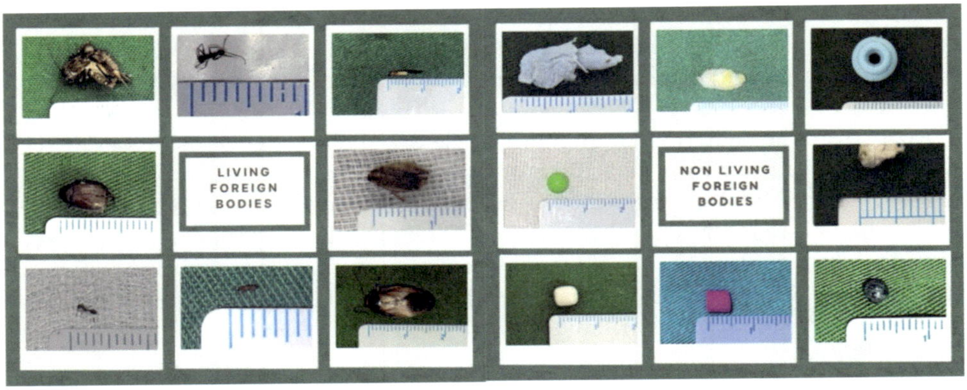

Figure 2.
Foreign bodies in the ear.

Animated or living foreign bodies must be removed dead to avoid the possibility that they will injure the ear canal when resisting during the extraction [17, 18]. Apart from that, there is also the possibility that insects will enter deeper into the ear canal.

For non-living foreign bodies, extraction can be carried out as soon as possible when it is discovered. They include sponge, eraser, paper, chalk, pencil tip and cotton wool [19].

5.2 Organic vs. inorganic

Organic foreign bodies are objects whose material comes from plants, while inorganic means the opposite. For most inorganic foreign bodies, management is not too urgent and needs to be done as soon as possible because it is hygroscopic, so it can absorb water and get bigger [20]. Batteries and other inorganic foreign objects are an exception, though. Traditionally, the most dangerous foreign object is a button battery, which has to be removed right away to prevent the surrounding soft tissue and bone from developing liquefactive necrosis. It is important to remember that a prolonged course of medication might worsen the effects of EAC edema and make the removal of foreign materials more challenging [20–22].

5.3 Metallic vs. non-metallic

Compared with other materials, metallic objects are better visualized through various imaging modalities, such as radiography and CT scans. In some cases of asymptomatic non-metallic foreign bodies, the foreign body appears the same in the surrounding soft tissue, both with and without the inflammatory process. Currently, magnetic methods are being used to remove metallic foreign objects, such as button batteries [16, 23, 24].

6. Clinical manifestations

6.1 Depend on the kind of foreign body

In living foreign bodies such as insects, intense irritation and pain can occur in the ear canal [10]. Furthermore, pruritus may accompany other problems. The patient typically complains of a fleeting bugging sensation, or the sensation that something is moving in their ear. Certain individuals typically have a history of neglected personal hygiene and have lived in unclean environments with verifiable insect infestations. This typically occurs while the patient is fast asleep. Numerous investigations have revealed that traveling outside the home is the source of bug foreign items detected in the ears. When a patient complains of an insect's foreign body, it usually happens rapidly and is obvious to them, so they go straight to emergency services and get help within hours [19, 25].

Meanwhile, non-animate foreign bodies can be asymptomatic. If the size of the foreign object is large enough, the complaint will cause a feeling of fullness in the ear. Other complaints can include otalgia and hearing loss [10, 19].

6.2 Depend on location of foreign body

The EAC is the most common location for ear foreign body cases [8]. Based on the material, complaints of foreign bodies in the EAC can vary, and can even be asymptomatic. Symptoms include otalgia, autorrhagia, unilateral ear discharge, hearing loss, tinnitus, cough, dizziness and facial muscle paresis. The complaints appear immediately, they are very disturbing and even so painful that patients are often immediately taken to the emergency department [8, 17].

In cases of foreign bodies in the middle ear, complaints usually occur due to perforation of the tympanic membrane that has previously formed [19, 26]. The most common cause of foreign items in the ear in patients with a history of chronic otitis media is ear picking, or in younger children, the habit of sticking objects into bodily cavities, including the ear. There have not been any reports of ear foreign bodies without a prior tympanic membrane perforation, albeit middle ear foreign body instances are quite uncommon.

According to a study of an 18-year-old child who was diagnosed with a middle ear foreign body, prominent clinical manifestations are intense pain in the neck and otorrhagia that resolves on its own. Particularly during the immediate post-traumatic phase, otorrhagia might happen. Hearing loss and recurring, unilateral chronic otorrhea are examples of further symptoms. The length of time the disease lasts determines how severe the symptoms are. If it has been too long, infection symptoms could manifest [26].

Foreign bodies lodged in the ear for a prolonged period often result in inflammatory reactions, sensitizing the external auditory canal and causing edema, which can make the removal process become more challenging [8].

7. Management

The kind of foreign body material and the area where the foreign body is still present determine how urgently cases of ear foreign bodies need to be handled. In addition, other factors that affect success include the doctor's skill, the equipment's accessibility, the patient's willingness to cooperate and the ease with which alien items can be visualized [9, 27]. Removal of the foreign body from the ear becomes contraindicated if these requirements are not satisfied. In addition to posing anatomical challenges to the EAC, the prior removal attempt's failure lowers patient cooperation [17, 28].

If prior attempts at ear foreign body removal are unsuccessful, the likelihood of the procedure needing to be performed in an operating room increases [13].

As a result, it has been decided from the beginning how many times the removal effort will be made and what method will be used if the first method fails. A general practitioner may try to remove irregular soft foreign bodies. In the interim, any hard, round, or soft, irregular foreign things that are not removed have to be directed to an Ear Nose and Throat (ENT) doctor. Furthermore, for greater success in removal, foreign objects with sharp edges or foreign things like batteries and vegetable material should be sent to an ENT Specialist [8, 14].

7.1 Instruments

7.1.1 Solid, non-compressible foreign body removal

Examples of solid, non-compressible foreign bodies to the ear include hair beads, toys, button batteries, food products and rocks.

- Removal by forceps

  Use forceps that can grasp the object's diameter if it is known to be a solid, non-compressible object. If the available forceps are unable to grab the object's diameter or be put along the object's periphery between the object and the external auditory canal, another method might work better [14, 16].

- Removal by cerumen loop

  A cerumen loop passing between the object and the Eustachian canal wall might be useful if the solid non-compressible object is small enough. To get behind the object and remove it from the ear, use the instrument's slightly inclined portion. This method could be especially helpful for solid, smooth materials that are slick or slippery [16].

- Removal by Frazier suction

  Applying a Frazier suction directly on the object is possible when it is coupled to a continuous low suction. To remove the patient's ear canal contents by suction, obstruct the insufflation port. It should be noted that the suction power might not be sufficient to remove the object [27].

- Removal by sterile swab stick with medical glue adhesive

  This approach includes use of a sterile swab: specifically the part of the swab without the cotton or rayon tip. Apply a tiny bit of medical adhesive glue to the swab's tip using the other end. This method could be especially helpful for extracting a spherical object that could be challenging to hold with forceps. Next, you can carefully and gently place the medical adhesive glue (cyanoacrylate) on the back of the swab stick directly on the object [27]. Take extreme care to avoid accidentally directing the glued end into the eustachian canal or pushing the foreign body farther into it [18]. Additionally, it is important to make sure that the applicator's tip is adhered to the foreign object rather than the EAC, which could lead to more damage or edema [17].

The foreign body at the end of the glued stick can be manually removed and removed as a single unit when the adhesive has dried after holding the glued end of the swab stick against the solid object for a short while [29].

7.1.2 Smooth foreign body removal

Example of smooth foreign bodies in the ear include cotton bud.

- Removal by Irrigation

  It is not advised to irrigate or syringe the ears, particularly when there are foreign items that contain elements like vegetables and batteries. Irrigation methods in vegetable matter allow the substance to swell and exacerbate the foreign object impaction [17]. Irrigation procedures applied to foreign items in batteries will result in liquefaction necrosis because the caustic contents of the battery will leak out. Additionally, foreign things (spongy objects) that expand as they absorb water should not be treated with irrigation techniques. In order to protect the tympanic membrane and EAC, management needs to happen more quickly [19].

A modified angiocatheter or butterfly catheter, with the needle, severed and the remaining portion attached to the syringe, is used in conjunction with a 20–30 cc syringe for ear syringing. In situations when there is a proven or suspected tympanic membrane hole, blind syringing should be avoided [17, 19]. The water used is at body temperature, neither too cold nor too hot [17]. Irrigation can generate vestibular stimulation, which can result in vertigo, nausea and vomiting if it is not at body temperature [27]. In order to get a clear view of the EAC, the pinna is retracted posteriorly and laterally. Next, water is sprayed into the EAC superiorly behind the foreign object until the water removes it [17].

7.2 Local or general anesthesia

Most ear foreign body extraction procedures are not performed under anesthesia. However, in some cases, such as pediatric populations and life-threatening complications, anesthesia is a consideration.

Local anesthesia is administered to reduce patient retrieval during removal. The use of local anesthesia is usually used in cases of living/animate insect foreign objects with the aim of killing the insect before extraction. The anesthetic used can be 1% lidocaine. Lidocaine is thought to have an irritating effect on insects, such as cockroaches, thereby encouraging insects to leave the EAC. However, local anesthesia is still not recommended in pediatric patients compared to general anesthesia due to its effectiveness in calming the patient. Apart from that, mineral oil, alcohol and olive oil can also be used to kill insects [15, 25, 27].

Meanwhile, the use of general anesthesia is indicated in cases of foreign objects that have been extracted but failed. General anesthesia can be given especially to aural foreign bodies in children that cannot be removed while the children are still conscious [9, 14]. General anesthesia is also indicated in cases of foreign bodies where the removal process is thought to be too complex. General anesthesia is expected to help facilitate better visualization and avoid injury during removal, especially due to instrumentation factors. If there are suspicions other than a foreign body, for example cholesteatoma or malignancy, an exploration procedure can be carried out under general anesthesia [29]. In addition, general anesthesia is used accidentally when a foreign object is discovered during other surgical procedures such as mastoidectomy for chronic otitis media and endoscopic sinus surgery for chronic sinusitis [15, 19].

7.3 Position

Before the patient is positioned for the removal process, first confirm the status of the tympanic membrane, whether it is still intact or there is a perforation. If intact, the patient can be asked to sit or lie down with the affected ear facing the examiner [18].

In children, one to two companions may be needed to ensure the child remains in place during removal without anesthesia. Pediatric patients can be seated on the parent's lap. The parent holds the child's body with one hand, and the other hand holds the patient's head; see **Figure 3**. The patient's head is positioned so that the affected ear faces the examiner, which provides good visualization. If the patient is lying down, either supine or prone, their head should be turned to improve access to the EAC. In children, it is important to examine the contralateral ear and other body orifices (e.g., nose) to rule out the presence of other foreign bodies [17].

7.4 Open surgery

Open surgery is usually performed in cases of foreign bodies in the middle ear. A case report shows a case of a middle ear foreign body in the form of silicone mold material from a hearing aid [30]. The eustachian tube, mastoid antrum and tympanic sinus all could contain these foreign items. Patients with stapedectomy via retroauricular approach owing to stapes footplate subluxation and partial fracture of the anterior half of the footplate were treated with canal wall up mastoidectomy, while other patients received treatment with transcanal foreign body removal, tympanoplasty and piston wire prosthesis insertion. Vestibular problems may arise as a result of the agent's toxicity to the cochleovestibular system. Therefore, individuals with external ear deformity, otorrhea, sudden hearing loss, dizziness, air-bone gap of more than 15 dB, cerumen impaction or otalgia should visit an ENT expert before having hearing aids installed. Another case report detailed a middle ear foreign body connected to radical mastoidectomy [29].

7.5 Antibiotics administration

In the context of attempting to remove a foreign object or because of the foreign object itself, the EAC is susceptible to get excoriation or laceration. Therefore, it

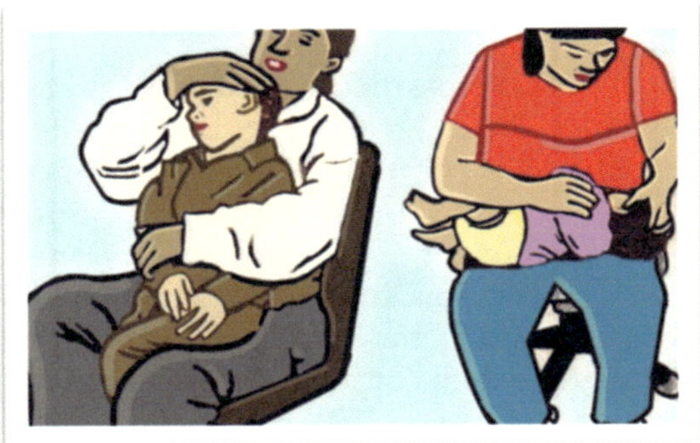

Figure 3.
How to hold child during the extraction procedure.

is necessary to assess the EAC before and after foreign body removal. Antibiotic ear drops may be considered in cases of lacerations or excoriations due to foreign bodies [18].

In a case report of a foreign insect body, ciprofloxacin ear drops were administered to prevent secondary infection. As a result, the tympanic membrane improved within 1 week of administering antibiotics [25].

In complaints that suggest the possibility of a cholesteatoma/granuloma as a reaction to a foreign body or other more severe infective causes, or complaints that have been treated with initial antibiotic therapy but have not improved, intravenous antibiotics can be considered, especially metronidazole and quinolones, then continued after the surgery [31].

8. Complications

Difficulties attempting to remove the foreign bodies could result in complications during extraction (tympanic membrane perforation, skin abrasion/laceration). When a patient attempts to remove a foreign body on their own after receiving first care from an emergency department physician, complications may arise. Documenting the ear canal both before and after treatment is crucial. The initial attempt to remove a foreign body is crucial since a failed removal will reduce the likelihood of success and may even raise the risk of complications. A referral is necessary if a foreign body, like a battery, is not removed; however, unless the patient is in discomfort, removal of the foreign body is not urgent. Patients treated by emergency department physicians and ENT experts have different levels of problems; patients treated by ENT specialists tend to have less issues. In order to lower the possibility of problems, emergency room physicians need to be aware of their capabilities and refer patients to ENT specialists.

Most complications secondary to aural foreign bodies documented in the current literature are mild and require no intervention such as lacerations to the ear canal or bleeding. In approximately 1% of instances, tympanic membrane perforations resulting from auditory foreign bodies are estimated to occur.

More severe complications show the patient having developed mastoiditis, suppurative labyrinthitis and necrotizing otitis externa secondary to aural foreign body dislodgement. These cases demonstrate the potentially destructive nature of aural foreign bodies due to the inflammatory response they can cause.

Author details

Jacky Munilson*, Yan Edward and Emilia Nissa Khairani
Andalas University, Padang, Indonesia

*Address all correspondence to: jackymunilson@yahoo.co.id

References

[1] Bansal M. Anatomy and physiology of ear. In: Bansal M, editor. Disease of Ear, Nose, and Throat. New Delhi: Jaypee Brothers Medical Publishers; 2013. pp. 1-26

[2] Dhingra PL, Dhingra S. Anatomy of ear. In: Dhingra PL, Dhingra S, editors. Diseases of Ear, Nose, and Throat & Head and Neck Surgery. 7th ed. New Delhi: RELX India Pvt. Ltd; 2018. pp. 3-14

[3] Snell RS. Mata dan Telinga. In: Suwahjo A, Liestyawan YA, editors. Anatomi Klinis Berdasarkan Sistem. Jakarta: EGC; 2011. pp. 626-636

[4] Liston SL, Duvall AJ. Embriologi, anatomi, dan fisiologi telinga. In: Effendi H, RAK S, editors. BOEIS Buku Ajar Penyakit THT. 6th ed. Jakarta: EGC; 1997. pp. 27-38

[5] Szymanski A, Geiger Z. Anatomy, head and neck, ear. In: StatPearls [Internet]. Treasure Island (FL): StatPearls Publishing; 2023. p. 2023. Available from: https://www.ncbi.nlm.nih.gov/books/NBK470359/ [Accessed: December 14, 2023]

[6] Eldahan MK, Abd El-Hady MR, Ibrahim HA. Effect of vagus nerve stimulation during ear wash. The Scientific Journal of Al-Azhar Medical Faculty, Girls. 2021;**5**(3):725-729. DOI: 10.4103/sjamf.sjamf_34_21

[7] Ghada MWF. Ear Anatomy. Global Journal of Otolaryngology. 2018;**4**(1):1-18

[8] Duan M, Morvil G, Badron J, Ganapathy S. Epidemiological trends and outcomes of children with aural foreign bodies in Singapore. Annals of the Academy of Medicine, Singapore. 2022;**51**:351-356

[9] Ponnuvelu K, Saniasiaya J, Gani NA. Intriguing aural foreign body and algorithm of management of foreign body. BML Case Reports. 2021;**14**:e24122

[10] Harini P, Kudamala S. Aural foreign bodies and their management: Our experience. International Journal of Otorhinolaryngology and Head and Neck Surgery. 2020;**6**:646-651

[11] Olajide TG, Ologe FE, Arigbede OO. Management of foreign bodies in the ear: A retrospective review of 123 cases in Nigeria. Ear, Nose, & Throat Journal. 2011;**90**(11):E16-E19

[12] Schuldt T, Grobmann W, Weiss NM, Ovari A, Mlynski R, Schraven SP. Aural and nasal foreign bodies in children. Epidemiology and correlation with hyperkinetic disorders, developmental disorder and congenital malformations. International Journal of Pediatric Otorhinolaryngology. 2019;**118**:165-9.q

[13] Xiao CC, Kshirsagar RS, Rivero A. Pediatric foreign bodies of the ear: A 10-year national analysis. International Journal of Pediatric Otorhinolaryngology. 2020;**138**:110354

[14] Prasad N, Harley E. The aural foreign body space: A review of pediatric ear foreign bodies and a management paradigm. International Journal of Pediatric Otorhinolaryngology. 2020;**132**:109871

[15] Shunyu NB, Akhtar H, Karim HM, Lyngdoh NM, Yunus M, Jamil M. Ear, nose, and throat foreign bodies removed under general anaesthesia: A Restrospective study. Journal of

Clinical and Diagnostic Research. 2017;**11**(2):MC01-MC04

[16] Craig SS, Cheek JA, Seith RW, West A. Removal of ENT foreign bodies in children. Emergency Medicine Australasia. 2015;**27**:145-147

[17] Davies PH, Benger JR. Foreign bodies in the nose and ear: A review of techniques for removal in the emergency department. Journal of Accident & Emergency Medicine. 2000;**17**(2):91-94

[18] Desai BK. Ear Foreign Body Removal. In: Ganti L, editor. Atlas of Emergency Medicine Procedures. Cham: Springer International Publishing; 2022. pp. 319-322

[19] Prasad KC, Sreelekshmi S, Abhilasha K, Anjali PK, Induvarsha G, Harshitha N. Unnoticed impacted foreign body ear presenting as chronic suppurative otitis media with postaural fistula: A rare case. International Journal of Otorhinolaryngology and Head and Neck Surgery. 2020;**6**:585-588

[20] Kim KH, Chung JH, Byun H, Zheng T, Jeong JH, Lee SH. Clinical characteristics of external Auditory Canal foreign bodies in children and adolescents. Ear, Nose, & Throat Journal. 2020;**99**(10):648-653

[21] Hernot S, Yadav SP, Kathuria B, Kaintura M. A rare complication due to button battery cell in ear. Indian Journal of Otology. 2016;**22**:52-55

[22] Premachandra DJ, McRae D. Severe tissue destruction in the ear caused by alkaline button batteries. Postgraduate Medical Journal. 1990;**66**:52-53

[23] Nivatvongs W, Ghabour M, Dhanasekar G. Difficult button battery ear foreign body removal: The magnetic solution. The Journal of Laryngology and Otology. 2015;**129**(1):93-94

[24] Scott RA, Wood C, Khan I. The novel use of a nasal bridle system to remove a foreign body in the ear. Clinical Case Reports. 2019;**7**:1439-1441

[25] Calleja T. 'A bugging feeling': A live foreign body in the ear. Archives of Disease in Childhood. 2020;**105**:689

[26] Elakhiri M, Ennouali A, Abdelfattah A, Darouassi Y, Ammar H. Foreign body of the middle ear: Case report and review of literature. Saudi Journal of Medicine. 2020;**5**(12):352-353

[27] Falcon-Chevere JL, Giraldez L, Rivera-Rivera JO, Suero-Salvador T. Critical ENT skills and procedures in the emergency department. Emergency Medicine Clinics of North America. 2013;**31**(1):29-58

[28] Schulze SL, Kerschner J, Beste D. Pediatric external auditory canal foreign bodies: A review of 698 cases. Otolaryngology and Head and Neck Surgery. 2002;**127**:73-78

[29] Shui-Hong Z, Qin-Ying W, Shen-Qing W. Middle ear foreign body causing cholesteatoma and external auditory canal granuloma: A case report. Journal of Otology. 2012;**7**(1):25-27

[30] Cho SD, Jang JH, Kim H, Cho YS, Kim Y, Koo JW, et al. Earmold foreign bodies in the middle ear necessitating surgical removal: Why otology specialists should screen candidates for hearing aids. Clinical and Experimental Otorhinolaryngology. 2021;**14**(2):235-239

[31] Woodley N, Slim MAM, Tikka T, Locke RR. Not 'just' a foreign body in the ear canal. BML Case Reports. 2019;**12**:e229302